T0338507

# LONG-TERM MANAGEMENT OF PATIENTS AFTER MYOCARDIAL INFARCTION

# DEVELOPMENTS IN CARDIOVASCULAR MEDICINE

Godfraind, T., Herman, A.S., Wellens, D., eds.: Entry blockers in cardiovascular and cerebral dysfunctions. ISBN 0-89838-658-6.
Morganroth, J., Moore, E.N., eds.: Interventions in the acute phase of myocardial infarction. ISBN 0-89838-659-4.
Abel, F.L., Newman, W.H., eds.: Functional aspects of the normal, hypertrophied, and failing heart. ISBN 0-89838-665-9.
Sideman, S., and Beyar, R., eds.: Simulation and imaging of the cardiac system. ISBN 0-89838-687-X.
van de Wall, E., Lie, K.I., eds.: Recent views on hypertrophic cardiomyopathy. ISBN 0-89838-694-2.
Beamish, R.E., Singal, P.K., Dhalla, N.S., eds.: Stress and heart disease. ISBN 0-89838-709-4.
Beamish, R.E., Panagia, V., Dhalla, N.S., eds.: Pathogenesis of stress-induced heart disease. ISBN 0-89838-710-8.
Morganroth, J., Moore, E.N., eds.: Cardiac arrhythmias: New therapeutic drugs and devices. ISBN 0-89838-716-7.
Mathes, P., ed.: Secondary prevention in coronary artery disease and myocardial infarction. ISBN 0-89838-736-1.
Stone, H. Lowell, Weglicki, W.B., eds.: Pathology of cardiovascular injury. ISBN 0-89838-743-4.
Meyer, J., Erbel, R., Rupprecht, H.J., eds.: Improvement of myocardial perfusion. ISBN 0-89838-748-5.
Reiber, J.H.C., Serruys, P.W., Slager, C.J.: Quantitative coronary and left ventricular cineangiography. ISBN 0-89838-760-4.
Fagard, R.H., Bekaert, I.E., eds.: Sports cardiology. ISBN 0-89838-782-5.
Reiber, J.H.C., Serruys, P.W., eds.: State of the art in quantitative coronary arteriography. ISBN 0-89838-804-X.
Roelandt, J., ed.: Color doppler flow imaging. ISBN 0-89838-806-6.
van de Wall, E.E., ed.: Noninvasive imaging of cardiac metabolism. ISBN 0-89838-812-0.
Liebman, J., Plonsey, R., Rudy, Y., eds.: Pediatric and fundamental electrocardiography. ISBN 0-89838-815-5.
Higler, H., Hombach, V., eds.: Invasive cardiovascular therapy. ISBN 0-89838-818-X.
Serruys, P.W., Meester, G.T., eds.: Coronary angioplasty: a controlled model for ischemia. ISBN 0-89838-819-8.
Tooke, J.E., Smaje, L.H., eds.: Clinical investigation of the microcirculation. ISBN 0-89838-833-3.
van Dam, Th., van Oosterom, A., eds.: Electrocardiographic body surface mapping. ISBN 0-89838-834-1.
Spencer, M.P., ed.: Ultrasonic diagnosis of cerebrovascular disease. ISBN 0-89838-836-8.
Legato, M.J., ed.: The stressed heart. ISBN 0-89838-849-X.
Safar, M.E., ed.: Arterial and venous systems in essential hypertension. ISBN 0-89838-857-0.
Roelandt, J., ed.: Digital techniques in echocardiography. ISBN 0-89838-861-9.
Dhalla, N.S., Singal, P.K., Beamish, R.E., eds.: Pathophysiology of heart disease. ISBN 0-89838-864-3.
Dhalla, N.S., Pierce, G.N., Beamish, R.E., eds.: Heart function and metabolism. ISBN 0-89838-865-1.
Dhalla, N.S., Innes, I.R., Beamish, R.E., eds.: Myocardial ischemia. ISBN 0-89838-866-X.
Beamish, R.E., Panagia, V., Dhalla, N.S., eds.: Pharmacological aspects of heart disease. ISBN 0-89838-867-8.
Ter Keurs, H.E.D.J., Tyberg, J.V., eds.: Mechanics of the circulation. ISBN 0-89838-870-8.
Sideman, S., Beyar, R., eds.: Activation metabolism and perfusion of the heart. ISBN 0-89838-871-6.
Aliot, E., Lazzara, R., eds.: Ventricular tachycardias. ISBN 0-89838-881-3.
Schneeweiss, A., Schettler, G.: Cardiovascular drug therapy in the elderly. ISBN 0-89838-883-X.
Chapman, J.V., Sgalambro, A., eds.: Basic concepts in doppler echocardiography. ISBN 0-89838-888-0.
Chien, S., Dormandy, J., Ernst, E., Matrai, A., eds.: Clinical hemorheology. ISBN 0-89838-807-4.
Morganroth, J., Moore, E. Neil, eds.: Congestive heart failure. ISBN 0-89838-955-0.
Heintzen, P.H., Bursch, J.H., eds.: Progress in digital angiocardiography. ISBN 0-89838-965-8.
Scheinman, M., ed.: Catheter ablation of cardiac arrhythmias. ISBN 0-89838-967-4.
Spaan, J.A.E., Bruschke, A.V.G., Gittenberger, A.C., eds.: Coronary circulation, ISBN 0-89838-978-X.
Bayes de Luna, A., ed.: Therapeutics in cardiology. ISBN 0-89838-981-X.

*This book is a volume in the series, "Advances in Myocardiology" (N.S. Dhalla, Series Editor).*
*"Advances in Myocardiology" is a subseries within "Developments in Cardiovascular Medicine".*

# LONG-TERM MANAGEMENT OF PATIENTS AFTER MYOCARDIAL INFARCTION

edited by

**C.T. Kappagoda**
**P.V. Greenwood**
*Department of Medicine*
*University of Alberta*
*Edmonton, Alberta, Canada*

Division of Cardiology
Department of Medicine
University of Alberta
Edmonton

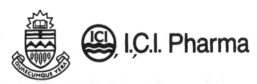

**Martinus Nijhoff Publishing**
*a member of the Kluwer Academic Publishers Group*
Boston/Dordrecht/Lancaster

**Distributors**

for North America: Kluwer Academic Publishers, 101 Philip Drive,
Assinippi Park, Norwell, MA 02061, USA

for the UK and Ireland: Kluwer Academic Publishers, MTP Press Limited,
Falcon House, Queen Square, Lancaster LA1 1RN, UK

for all other countries: Kluwer Academic Publishers Group, Distribution
Centre, Post Office Box 322, 3300 AH Dordrecht, The Netherlands

**Library of Congress Cataloging-in-Publication Data**

Long-term management of patients after myocardial
  infarction.

  (Developments in cardiovascular medicine)
  Includes bibliographies.
    1. Heart—Infarction—Patients—Rehabilitation.
2. Coronary heart disease—Patients—Rehabilitation.
I. Kappagoda, C. T.  II. Greenwood, P. V.  III. Series.
[DNLM: 1. Myocardial Infarction—rehabilitation.
2. Long Term Care.  W1 DE997VME / WG 300 L848]
RC685.I6L66  1987          616.1 '2406          87-28207
ISBN 0-89838-352-8

*We dedicate this book to our patients.*

# CONTENTS

viii

## IV. FUTURE TRENDS

## PREFACE

The management of patients who present with a myocardial infarction has altered radically over the past two decades. The expansion of knowledge relating to the epidemiology of the condition together with a greater understanding of the causes of the early mortality from it have resulted in major changes in the way these patients are treated during the acute phase of the illness. The development of 'dedicated' Coronary Care Units in hospitals and the recognition of the need for 'Mobile Coronary Care Units' in the community have made a major impact upon the early mortality from myocardial infarction.

Over the past decade, a great deal of attention has been paid to strategies designed to limit the size of a myocardial infarct. As an extension of this approach, the 1980's have seen the evolution of techniques for revascularization of ischemic tissue. All these procedures while appearing to hold the promise of reducing the acute mortality from myocardial infarction, create the need for a planned approach to the long term management of these patients. While there are some modest indications that coronary atherosclerosis could be arrested or even reversed, for all practical purposes it remains a chronic progressive disease. Thus there is an increasing need to blend the traditional approaches to the rehabilitation of these patients with the therapeutic interventions which are being developed for the 'in-hospital' phase of the illness. In this volume we have attempted to do so by bringing together the views of individuals who have made important contributions to our knowledge of the various aspects of the long-term management of patients recovering from myocardial infarction.

We feel that this book should be of value to both physicians and non-physicians who are involved in the follow up care and rehabilitation of patients after acute myocardial infarction.

Although some of the chapters deal with more specialized aspects of cardiac care and will be of special interest to cardiologists, the majority of the book should enable the general readers to get a better perspective on present management and prepare them to appreciate future developments in this rapidly evolving area.

We wish to acknowledge a huge debt of gratitude to our secretaries, Mrs. Sharon Campbell and Mrs. Erin Gardner who have coped with all of the many problems in the production of this book and prepared the final drafts of the manuscripts. In doing all this they have managed to continue smiling and run the rest of the office with much appreciated efficiency.

Finally, we would like to thank I.C.I. Pharma and Martinus Nijhoff Publishing who have maintained their support for us in this venture.

# LONG-TERM MANAGEMENT OF PATIENTS AFTER MYOCARDIAL INFARCTION

# 1

## INTRODUCTION: LONG-TERM MANAGEMENT OF PATIENTS AFTER MYOCARDIAL INFARCTION

N. K. Wenger

Emory University School of Medicine, Atlanta, Georgia, USA

The initial chapters of this monograph present the background epidemiologic data that can help guide recommendations for the long-term management of patients after myocardial infarction; the authors address the changing patterns of atherosclerotic coronary heart disease, specifically targeting the prehospital, hospital and posthospital aspects of coronary mortality. The varied methodologies used to assess functional status after myocardial infarction are reviewed in the following section; this functional assessment forms the basis for choosing among the medical and surgical therapeutic options delineated in the subsequent section. Medical interventions, in addition to pharmacotherapy, include coronary risk reduction, exercise training, and psychological counselling and guidance. Contemporary indications are reviewed for both coronary angioplasty and coronary surgery. A final section explores potential future concepts for management, expansions of our therapeutic armamentarium that are likely to be available within the next decade.

## CHANGING PATTERNS OF CORONARY ARTERY DISEASE AND SURVIVAL AFTER MYOCARDIAL INFARCTION

The striking decrease in coronary mortality in the U.S. and in several other nations during the past two decades was largely unanticipated. Although coronary heart disease mortality continues to decrease in many countries of the world, controversy persists as to the relative contributions of a variety of factors: primary preventive efforts; decreasing severity of coronary disease; availability of bystander CPR and improved emergency transport facilities and services; better hospital care, including the contributions of intensive coronary care and newer medical and surgical therapies; and advances in posthospital care, encompassing a variety of medical therapies and rehabilitation and secondary prevention programs.

Labarthe challenges the thesis that a decrease in the incidence of coronary heart disease relates to primary preventive efforts, whereas a decrease in case fatality after infarction reflects improved medical care. He suggests that a reduction in coronary incidence may be influenced by the medical management of hypertension or by coronary bypass surgery, whereas coronary risk reduction may improve survival even following a recognized myocardial infarction. In the nine epidemiologic studies of postinfarction survival reviewed, Labarthe focuses attention on the differences in population size, in age range, in criteria for the diagnosis of infarction, and in the starting point of observation of the patients, whether at hospital admission or at hospital discharge. In general, a decrease of 20-30% in early mortality has been observed (except among younger subjects), with little change evident in late survival (except in the Goteborg study, where the improvement in posthospital survival was attributed to the widespread use of beta blocking drugs). Thus, whereas medical care may have favorably affected the early postinfarction mortality, it appears to have had little impact on long-term survival, save for the effect of beta blocker therapy just cited. These dynamic changes in the natural history of coronary heart disease define several important research needs: (1) the delineation of changes in the population within which cases of myocardial infarction occur, (2) the description of changes in the population who experience and survive myocardial infarction, and (3) the characterization of modifications achieved by preventive measures and by treatment of recognized disease.

Kappagoda's presentation focuses on the changing trends in prehospital and hospital mortality, with emphasis on the differences in data obtained from community surveys, from those relating to hospital admissions and discharges, and even those derived from patients referred to tertiary care institutions. In general, the overall mortality of patients hospitalized for an initial infarction in North American centers prior to 1950 was approximately 20%. Nearly 70% of the deaths from a first infarction occurred within the initial 24 hours, provided that patients were hospitalized within the first 6 hours of illness. Indeed, the majority of deaths occurred within the first several hours after the onset of symptoms. Despite a lack of objective data, coronary care units were considered to have contributed to the overall decline in ischemic heart disease mortality in the United States because of the lack of significant changes in the risk factor profile of the population during that period and because of the lack of impact of coronary bypass surgery during the late 1960s and early 1970s. There was also supporting evidence that the rapid provision of emergency coronary care by mobile units and the prompt institution of cardiopulmonary resuscitation might reduce subsequent hospital mortality. Thus, in circumstances where coronary care units are supplemented by mobile coronary care facilities, a 12-15% hospital mortality from myocardial infarction can currently be anticipated in patients younger than age 70 years. A further change in the mode of postinfarction mortality is that arrhythmia-related deaths have declined, whereas the mechanical consequences of cardiac failure and myocardial rupture have increased in importance as contributors to fatality.

Norris' assessment, based primarily on data from the Auckland, New Zealand hospitals, suggests that better inhospital care, rather than a decrease in the severity of coronary disease, should be credited for the improvement in survival, particularly the improved management of arrhythmias, shock, and congestive cardiac failure. He suggests that, although beta blockade (by decreasing myocardial oxygen demand) may improve the prognosis following infarction, even better outcomes should be anticipated to result from reperfusion therapies such as acute thrombolysis and/or coronary angioplasty. Norris offers that a further improvement in outcome is likely to be attained as a result of extensive public education regarding the need for early response to coronary symptoms, and an improved acute care transport system, with more efficient entry into the hospital intensive care setting; all these aspects may enable earlier reperfusion therapies. He identifies late mortality as related predominantly to older age, cardiac enlargement, and increased severity of the congestive cardiac failure. Indeed, the severity of the left ventricular dysfunction appears far more predictive than the severity of the coronary atherosclerotic obstruction in determining an adverse prognosis. A patent infarct-related artery appears to correlate with an improved outlook; the residual left ventricular dysfunction is far less severe, possibly owing to spontaneous reperfusion. Since left ventricular dysfunction is the major determinant of an adverse prognosis, the author suggests that left ventricular end systolic volume, rather than end diastolic volume or ejection fraction, provides the greatest predictive accuracy in regard to outcome. Long-term survival after infarction, during the period following discharge from hospital, may also be improving.

## ASSESSMENT OF FUNCTION FOLLOWING MYOCARDIAL INFARCTION
### Physiology of Exercise: Cardiovascular Responses

Shepherd and Shepherd from the Mayo Clinic describe the normal physiologic responses to exercise as the basis for understanding the exercise-dependent tests used to assess functional status following myocardial infarction. They describe a complex interaction of local and humoral adjustments of the heart and of the resistance and capacitance vessels to meet the metabolic demands of physical activity. They delineate the anticipated differences in response to supine and upright exercise, as well as changes in response to exercise that are associated with heart failure.

### Noninvasive Evaluation of Ventricular Function

Because of the pivotal role of postinfarction ventricular function previously noted, Noble and associates discuss the noninvasive approaches to measuring ventricular function following myocardial infarction. Exercise studies of ventricular function are complicated by the potential adverse effects of the resultant ischemia on ventricular function; thus the authors prefer to evaluate ventricular function at rest. Although radionuclide-based studies of the left ventricular blood pool provide optimal definition of the left ventricular ejection fraction, the special facilities and equipment required to perform these tests prohibit their being considered a routine measurement technique for office practice. The authors believe that transcutaneous Doppler determination of aortic blood flow velocity offers promise for noninvasively evaluating resting left ventricular function.

Exercise Testing, Exercise Radionuclide Studies & Risk Stratification

Chaitman's discussion of exercise testing after myocardial infarction addresses the role of this procedure in identifying patients at high risk of recurrent coronary events; this risk stratification is designed to select those patients who require early coronary arteriography in consideration for urgent coronary angioplasty or coronary bypass graft surgery. Abnormalities at exercise testing that suggest this high-risk status include ST segment depression at low levels of exercise, the inability to exercise beyond an intensity of 4 Mets, the inability to increase the exercise systolic blood pressure $> 110$ mmHg or exercise-induced hypotension, and the occurrence of exercise-induced ventricular tachycardia. When radionuclide studies are coupled with exercise testing, reversible Thallium perfusion defects, increased Thallium lung uptake, a fall in the exercise ejection fraction, and new exercise-related wall motion abnormalities also have adverse prognostic significance. Conversely, patients who can complete the low-level predischarge exercise test without abnormalities have a favorable prognosis. Exercise-induced angina often predicts postinfarction angina and increases the likelihood of unstable angina, recurrent infarction, and the need for subsequent coronary bypass graft surgery. When angiography is not routinely performed after thrombolytic therapy has been administered, the application of exercise testing for prognostic risk stratification is appropriate to help select patients who require early coronary angiography and the use of myocardial revascularization techniques vs those who are best treated by pharmacologic means. Chaitman suggests that most patients who develop greater than one millimeter of exercise-induced ST depression at low-level exercise (less than 4 Mets) should be considered for coronary angiography.

## Exercise Echocardiography

Crawford summarizes the emerging role of exercise echocardiography following myocardial infarction. Because exercise-induced or intensified abnormalities indicate a high likelihood of future cardiac events, and because delineation of areas of myocardial asynergy distant from the site of infarction suggests multivessel coronary disease, noninvasive means of identifying these features are highly desirable. The author reports a high incidence of satisfactory two-dimensional echocardiographic images at rest and following low-level treadmill exercise in patients in the early postinfarction period; the experience of the San Antonio, Texas Veterans Adminitration Hospital Group suggests that the results of exercise echocardiography in detecting exercise-induced wall motion abnormalities are comparable to those obtained using radionuclide imaging after upright bicycle exercise. The lesser requirements for elaborate equipment and facilities render echocardiographic studies a more feasible means of detecting abnormalities of ventricular function, both those present at rest and those induced by exercise. Crawford considers that Doppler flow velocity measurements may provide added information; based on 2-D echocardiographic estimation of aortic area, Doppler measurements of aortic flow velocity can be used to estimate stroke volume; aortic flow velocity acceleration can provide information about the left ventricular function status. Many patients have wall motion abnormalities at rest following myocardial infarction. Worsening of wall motion abnormalities with exercise or the appearance of new exercise-induced wall motion abnormalities has adverse implications for prognosis. Wall motion abnormalities in areas of myocardium remote from the infarction suggest multivessel coronary disease. Echocardiographic imaging thus appears to provide additive information to that derived from the exercise ECG, helping to identify patients with ventricular dysfunction in addition to those with exercise-induced abnormalities compatible with myocardial ischemia.

## Coronary Arteriography

Horgan reviews the advantages and limitations of coronary arteriography, emphasizing its changing role relative to newer acute approaches to myocardial revascularization; thrombolysis, coronary angioplasty, and early coronary bypass graft surgery. Coronary arteriography is indicated during the early hospital phase of infarction to determine candidacy for intracoronary thrombolysis, with or without subsequent angioplasty; or candidacy for early coronary bypass surgery (during the initial 4-6 hours after infarction). Arteriography is also warranted after intravenous thrombolysis in patients hospitalized later than 4-6 hours following infarction, in those who manifest unstable angina during the hospitalization, or in those who develop mitral regurgitation or clinical evidence of ventricular septal defect (septal rupture). Indications for coronary arteriography during the convalescent phase of myocardial infarction are often determined by the results of the noninvasive studies designed to stratify patients by risk status; high-risk characteristics that warrant arteriography include angina pectoris at rest or at low-level activity, ischemia induced during low levels of exercise, heart failure with a persistently reduced ejection fraction, high-grade ventricular arrhythmias in the presence of a reduced ejection fraction, and non-Q-wave myocardial infarction.

## THERAPEUTIC OPTIONS FOLLOWING MYOCARDIAL INFARCTION
### Beta Blockade

Greenwood's assessment of the role of beta adrenoreceptor blocking drugs in patients with myocardial infarction is based on data derived from more than 20 large clinical trials; of importance is the large variety of beta blocking agents that were used and the widely differing times following myocardial infarction when beta blockade was instituted. The potential advantages of beta blocking therapy, both administered acutely and on a chronic basis, include a decrease in myocardial oxygen demand, a decrease in size of the infarction, limitation of arrhythmias, and favorable antiplatelet effects. Potential disadvantages are the occurrence of bradyarrhythmias (including complete heart block), congestive heart failure, and hypotension; as well as a variety of symptomatic side effects. Although the results of several trials suggest that beta blocking therapy improves survival, extrapolation of these data to older and higher-risk patients is questionable, and the cost of beta blockade is significant. It has been suggested that cessation of smoking by only half of all patients who continue to smoke cigarettes following infarction can effect the same improvement in survival without significant cost. The duration of benefit of beta blocking therapy is also uncertain. Greenwood appropriately notes that many strategies used in the contemporary management of patients with myocardial infarction were not available during most beta blocking drug trials, specifically the newer myocardial revascularization procedures. Risk stratification, as noted above, may offer the possibility of selecting the moderate to high risk patients who would be more likely to benefit from intensive interventions. Greenwood cautions against the routine widespread adoption of beta blocking therapy as the major secondary preventive approach in patients with myocardial infarction.

## Coronary Angioplasty

Based on information from the NHLBI-PTCA Registry, Bourassa and coauthors concluded that PTCA should be performed during the acute phase of myocardial infarction to recanalize the infarct-related artery. As previously noted, preservation of left ventricular function is a major favorable prognostic sign; thus early (within 6 hours after infarction) PTCA of the infarct-related artery is indicated to restore blood flow and to preserve left ventricular function. Delayed PTCA should not be undertaken in most patients during the evolutionary phase of myocardial infarction because the procedure entails an increased risk and offers little or no advantage. Once the infarct has stabilized, during the convalescent phase, PTCA is again appropriate to relieve the residual stenosis in the infarct-related artery, as well as to treat additional lesions if multivessel coronary disease is present. Data are not available that compare the results of isolated PTCA with the results of thrombolysis followed by PTCA. The frequent residual significant coronary obstruction following successful thrombolysis often requires coronary angioplasty or bypass graft surgery for improvement in left ventricular function to occur. Multilesion and multivessel PTCA may be undertaken to achieve myocardial revascularization during the convalescent phase of infarction. Although, based on the NHLBI-PTCA Registry data, significant relief of angina follows successful PTCA, restenosis of the dilated arteries is frequent, particularly during the first year of follow-up. This occurrence often mandates either repeated angioplasty or urgent coronary bypass surgery. Comparison of outcomes of PTCA and coronary bypass graft surgery in patients eligible for both procedures is currently under investigation.

## Coronary Bypass Surgery; Laser Endarterectomy

Keon and Koshal's discussion of elective coronary bypass surgery after myocardial infarction reemphasizes the independent determinants of adverse outcome during the initial year following infarction: left ventricular dysfunction, residual myocardial ischemia, ventricular arrhythmias, and triple vessel coronary disease. Patients with these high-risk characteristics appear to derive the greatest benefit from myocardial revascularization; and laser endarterectomy is suggested to increase the likelihood of successful revascularization in patients with significant distal vessel disease. Other surgical procedures considered after infarction include left ventricular aneurysmectomy for patients with symptomatic manifestations, particularly angina pectoris or life-threatening cardiac arrhythmias, subendocardial resection or cryoablation therapy for reentrant tachyarrhythmias unresponsive to medical therapy; and cardiac transplantation for selected patients with end stage coronary disease.

## Coronary Risk Reduction

Although the severity of the infarction is the main determinant of early postinfarction mortality, Puska asserts that cigarette smoking, hypertension, diabetes mellitus, physical inactivity, and elevated LDL cholesterol levels predict reinfarction and coronary death during long-term follow-up. He emphasizes the potential benefits of risk reduction, citing little hazard and limited costs Major emphasis should be devoted to cessation of smoking, control of hypertension, and weight reduction as evidence for the efficacy of supervised exercise and of lipid-lowering remains limited. Puska advocates a behavioral approach to risk reduction that includes provision of information, persuasion to adopt health-related behaviors, training in the skills needed for the adoption of favorable behaviors, and provision of social support and environmental modification to reinforce health habits. The important roles of a variety of health professionals in risk reduction are cited.

## Exercise Training

Pollock reviews the effects of physical activity on coronary mortality, as evident in data derived from nine secondary prevention trials. Two trials showed a favorable effect and seven had inconclusive results; the favorable studies, however, involved multiple risk reduction in addition to exercise training. Pooled data from all nine trials, however, showed a significant benefit of exercise. Thus, although exercise may favorably alter coronary risk by increasing HDL cholesterol, reducing blood pressure, and encouraging other favorable lifestyle alterations, a multifactorial program of coronary risk reduction is judged optimal. Most patients who exercise following infarction improve their functional capacity, with primarily peripheral adaptations evident during low- to moderate-intensity exercise programs. A combination of peripheral and central adaptations are reported to result from high-intensity, long-term exercise training regimens; the latter, though, may entail a greater risk of intercurrent cardiovascular events. Pollock suggests stratification of myocardial infarction patients into high- and low-risk subgroups; high-risk patients with medical instability are recommended to undergo more conservative and cautious exercise training.

## Psychologic Management

Mayou delineates the threefold importance of psychologic aspects of management of patients after myocardial infarction to (1) minimize the psychosocial consequences of the illness, (2) effect compliance with recommendations for care, and (3) contribute to behavioral changes as part of secondary prevention. Provision of information, and explanations and counselling are suggested to alleviate the anxiety and depression of the acute illness; and a rehabilitative approach is advocated to facilitate rapid return to the preillness family, social, work, sexual and leisure activities. Physical activity regimens are advised, but no advantages appear to derive from structured, supervised exercise programs. Support, encouragement, and reassurance are among the benefits of group educational and physical activities; individual counselling may be beneficial as well. The value of tailoring a rehabilitative approach to the specific needs of each patient is cited, with additional selective treatment recommended for particular problems: risk reduction, physical activity, return to work, sexual activity, family problems, etc. Mayou highlights the comparable needs of patients recovering from coronary bypass surgery.

## TRENDS FOR FUTURE INTERVENTIONS AFTER MYOCARDIAL INFARCTION
### Calcium Channel Blocking Therapy

Nayler and associates discuss the potential role of calcium channel blocking drugs in the long-term management of patients with ischemic heart disease. Whereas improvement in long-term outcome has been described with the use of beta adrenoreceptor antagonists and platelet inhibitor drugs, most clinical trials of calcium channel blockers have not had a comparable favorable effect; the notable exception is the study of diltiazem in patient with non-Q-wave infarction where a short-term protective effect was demonstrated against reinfarction. The authors cite this as evidence that calcium channel blockers may protect potentially jeopardized myocardium in appropriate situations. Citing subset data from other clinical trials of calcium blocking agents, the premise is developed that this category of drugs can reduce or delay ischemic injury if used prophylactically, with an adequate drug concentration available prior to an ischemic episode; this condition can currently be met by the available long-acting slow calcium channel blockers. The major posturaled mechanism of benefit relates to the attenuation of reperfusion-induced calcium overload that results in energy-depletion, membrane disruption, platelet aggregation, and coronary vasoconstriction, to name a few adverse consequences of calcium overload. Further, the authors suggest that the calcium channel blocking drug effect of depleting myocardial norepinephrine may limit the ischemia-precipitated release of endogenous norepinephrine and its deleterious consequences. Slow calcium channel blocker therapy has also been shown to attenuate atherosclerotic plaque formation and possibly to hasten its regression, as well as to slow the smooth muscle cell proliferation that is part of the atherosclerotic process. Coronary vasodilatation is another potential favorable effect of calcium channel blockers.

In summary, then, the authors postulate that the benefit of slow calcium channel blockade in the long-term management of patients with coronary heart disease necessitates long-term prophylactic therapy; this approach may limit the progression and reduce the intensity of a subsequent ischemic episode.

Antilipidemic Drug Therapy

Packard and Shepherd address the importance of specific membrane protein "receptors" for cholesterol-containing lipoproteins in the blood in modulating the intracellular intake of circulating sterols, thus regulating the balance between intracellular and extracellular sterol concentrations. The liver is the most important site for lipoprotein synthesis and secretion, and contains about 70% of human LDL receptor activity. The relative concentrations of cholesterol in liver, blood and peripheral tissues appear regulated by a variety of specific protein receptors that permit cholesterol entry or extract the sterol from tissue cells; the function of these protein receptors may be altered by pharmacotherapy. Homozygous individuals with familial hypercholesterolemia cannot maintain the correct balance between hepatic and circulating cholesterol. Administration of sequestrant resins such as cholestyramine or colestipol to heterozygous patients can lower circulating LDL; by removing bile acids from the circulation, it can potentially increase hepatic LDL receptor activity, causing LDL extraction from the circulation; however, endogenous hepatic cholesterologenesis blunts the effectiveness of this therapy. The newer hypocholesterolemic agents such as compactin and mevinolin, designed to inhibit cholesterol synthesis by inhibiting HMG CoA reductase, the rate-limiting enzyme, may prevent the secondary rise in cholesterol synthesis and further increase LDL receptor activity. In patients with type III hyperlipoproteinemia with defective plasma clearance of chylomicrons and VLDL remnants, estrogen administration may reduce the remnant accumulation by stimulating hepatic lipoprotein receptor activity. A further potential favorable therapy could involve the transfer of sterol between the plasma and tissue cholesterol pools, most probably by altering intracellular cholesterol esterification; agents that inhibit cholesterol esterification in animals by blocking acyl Coenzyme A: cholesterol acyltransferase (ACAT) can improve cholesterol excretion by upgrading HDL receptor activity; this aspect has not yet been addressed in humans. Thus, pharmacotherapy capable of altering membrane receptor activity may potentially favorably affect tissue cholesterol levels and retard or reduce atherogenesis.

## Platelet-influencing Agents; Antithrombotic Therapy

Ritter offers a third area for potential favorable pharmacotherapeutic intervention, that related to the roles of thromboxane $A_2$ and prostacycline ($PGI_2$) in platelet-blood vessel interactions. The six published trials of aspirin use in patients with myocardial infarction indicate a significant improvement in recurrence-free survival; comparable results have been reported from trials of aspirin given to patients with transient ischemic attacks and with unstable angina. The current dominating thesis is that the clinical antithrombotic effect of aspirin is due to its inhibition of platelet thromboxane $A_2$ production; however, there is much interest in selective inhibition of platelet cyclo-oxygenase, sparing vascular cyclo-oxygenase; low-dose aspirin is currently the most feasible agent for this intervention. No studies using low-dose (presumably platelet-selective) aspirin have yet been reported; data from the low-dose aspirin trials currently in progress are likely to further elucidate the mechanism(s) of the antithrombotic effects of aspirin. Thromboxane synthase inhibitors are currently being tested in animal models; if effective, these agents, combined with thromboxane receptor antagonists, may exert potent antithrombotic effects.

The foregoing serve to highlight several areas where advances in pharmacotherapy may improve the outlook of medically-managed patients following myocardial infarction. They are likely to be equally applicable to the long-term care of patients who have undergone surgical myocardial revascularization.

# I.  PATTERNS OF CORONARY ARTERY DISEASE AND SURVIVAL

# 2

CHANGING PATTERNS IN THE EPIDEMIOLOGY OF CORONARY ARTERY DISEASE:
TRENDS IN SURVIVAL AFTER MYOCARDIAL INFARCTION

Darwin R. Labarthe

The Epidemiology Research Center, The School of Public Health, The
University of Texas Health Science Center at Houston, Houston, Texas

## BACKGROUND

Patterns in the epidemiology of coronary artery disease (or
coronary heart disease, CHD) are doubtless changing continually in
many ways, only some of which are recognized at any given time. In
the entire history of the epidemiology of CHD, perhaps no such change
has been more prominent than the striking decrease in mortality
observed in the United States as a whole over the past two decades
and in several other countries at roughly the same time.

As a result, the topic of "changing patterns" has been dominated
in recent years by interest in this phenomenon. Having occurred
without prediction, its explanation has been elusive (1,2). This is
due in part to the theoretical plausibility of a number of
explanations which could be complementary as well as competing
hypotheses, and none of which has been conclusively established or
rejected on the available evidence. In addition, the issue has
frequently been oversimplified by reference to "the decline" as
though a uniform process were affecting the entire population of the
U.S. and other countries with similar mortality trends.

The epidemiologic research stimulated by this interest has led
to the analysis of secular trends in mortality data for many areas of
the world, from single localities to multinational comparisons. As a
result, important variations in the recent changes in CHD mortality
have been recognized, both within and between countries (3,4,5,6). A
single explanation of such diverse changes may be an inappropriate
expectation.

A long-range objective of research on this problem has been to distinguish between two aspects of the natural history of CHD, incidence (or the occurrence of new cases of disease) and mortality (death from the disease), or more restrictively case-fatality (or the proportion of cases dying in some arbitrarily defined time interval). This distinction has often been reduced to the simplistic formulation that a decrease in incidence measures the effects of reduction in specific risk factors for CHD, while a decrease in case-fatality after the occurrence of acute myocardial infarction (MI) measures the effects of medical care: Primary prevention is reflected wholly and exclusively in incidence, and the corresponding relation holds between medical care and case-fatality.

The limitations of this view are apparent when the potential for overlapping effects is taken into account: Medical care in the absence of overt MI includes such interventions as management of high blood pressure and coronary bypass surgery, while reduction in risk factors may plausibly improve the prognosis for survival even though a recognized MI was not prevented. Thus incidence may be influenced by medical care and survival by early, though insufficient, improvements in risk factors. The separate effects of these types of influences may be only partly distinguishable without direct assessment of risk factor and medical care experience of the population studied.

Nonetheless, the recent epidemiologic literature includes not only the large number of reports concerning mortality trends already alluded to but also a few on incidence and, most relevant here, several which address the issue of survival after MI. From the perspective of this literature as a whole, the latter studies are of most immediate importance because they deal with the population which has experienced an MI but survived, those for whom long-term management after MI is possible. Among the many questions which might be raised about this population, the studies of survival after MI address especially the following:

1. Have there been demonstrable trends in the proportions of MI cases surviving, either short- or long-term?

2. Are there consistencies in such trends within or between studies of distinct subgroups or populations?

3. How have the investigators interpreted their observations, with respect particularly to the possible effects of medical care on survival after MI or, by extension, on trends in CHD mortality?

In the sections which follow, the reports on survival after MI will be examined in some detail and the answers to these questions determined. It will then be possible, in conclusion, to consider the broader question of changing patterns in survival after MI and some of their implications for long-term treatment of this very large and important target population.

## STUDIES OF SURVIVAL AFTER MI:  DESIGN AND METHODS

Nine epidemiologic studies which address trends in post-MI survival are described in Table I (7-16). The populations studied were predominantly geographically defined in urban localities, although two health insurance groups and one employee population were studied as well. The reports were published within the past decade and presented data for calendar periods or time intervals of from 5 or 6 to more than 30 years, mainly during the 1960s and 1970s. (Years shown in the Table do not reflect the sometimes extended follow up of cohorts still being defined in the latest year shown.)

Population sizes are given for studies where they were reported, often including population estimates at both starting and ending dates of the study. The adult age range, beginning in the 20s and 30s, was represented in all studies, but there were potentially important differences in the upper age limit, from as low as 59 years of age in Goteborg (No. 6) to no upper limit in 2 or 3 of the studies (Nos. 1,3 and 9). Both men and women were included in all studies except No. 4, although the numbers of events in women were often too few for separate analysis.

The conditions selected for review in the present report included acute myocardial infarction in all instances, and this class of events is the central focus of attention. However, the studies differed importantly in the categorization of conditions, such that sudden unexpected death (SUD) was in some instances distinguished from MI generally. In particular, the Rochester study (No. 3) presented data separately for SUD and MI as first manifestations of

CHD, while those in Auckland and the Du Pont employees (Nos. 7 and 8) included SUD in the MI category without differentiation. In the Minneapolis-St. Paul study (No. 5), the most detailed classification of events by time and location of occurrence was given, with distinction between out-of-hospital, emergency room and hospital ward deaths; only the in-hospital (post-emergency room) events are addressed here. Criteria for the diagnosis of MI differed among studies as well and could not always be interpreted unambiguously from the published information; the original reports and their cross-references should be consulted for details.

Generally large numbers of MI cases were available for study. These numbers are presented either for the overall period of study (e.g., 1307 cases in Baltimore for two study periods combined) or for discrete time periods (e.g., 288 cases in a 40% population sample and 876 cases in complete coverage of the population of Auckland, in 1974 and 1981, respectively).

These studies differ importantly in the approach to assessment of survival after MI. Appreciation of the differences may be aided by consideration of the starting point of observation of each case, the definitions adopted for the various periods of survival, and the nature of the trends examined. These final descriptors in Table 1 require some comment for each study, based on interpretation of the methods of study as presented in each publication.

In Baltimore, hospital admission was the first point of departure for monitoring of in-hospital deaths, with separate presentation of data for all admissions and for those surviving at least 24, or 48, hours in hospital. Second, hospital discharge was taken as the start of observation, with follow up reported for periods from 6 to 10 years after discharge. Both types of survival experience, in- and post-hospital, were simply compared for the two cohorts formed in the respective 12-month periods, mid-1966 to mid-1967 and calendar 1971 (7).

The Kaiser-Permanente study was quite briefly reported and presented the proportions of deaths among hospitalized MI patients, by calendar year, over the consecutive years from 1971-1977. (The numbers of patients were not reported.)

For Rochester, MN, the original report of 1981 and the extension in 1986 provided information on all new CHD cases identified, presumably as of the time of diagnosis rather than hospital admission. Thus SUD, the separately accounted for as deaths within 24 hours of onset of the event, included out-of-hospital deaths. The start of observation for the subsequent intervals studied -- from 1-30 days, from onset to 5 years, and from 31 days to as long as 10 years -- was apparently the date of diagnosis as well. Short-term survival was described as the average for the cohort of each successive 5-year (or most recently 4-year) calendar period, and survival curves were estimated to 10 years after 30 days of survival for the 1965-1969 and the 1970-1974 cohorts (9,10).

In the HIP study, patients who attended a baseline examination within 12 months of discharge from the hospital for treatment of MI were followed for up to 4 or 5 years to estimate post-hospital survival. The average survival curve for patients entering in the 1960s was compared with that for patients entering in the 1970s (11).

As noted earlier, the relation of time and setting to early mortality in MI cases was examined in detail by the investigators in the Minneapolis-St. Paul study. Most nearly comparable with other available data were those selected for inclusion here, beginning with hospital (as distinct from emergency room) admission and ending with death or hospital discharge. The resulting mortality rates were compared between the two study periods, calendar 1970 and 1980 (12).

The data presented for the MI cases in Goteborg, Sweden, were based on records of live hospital discharges and follow up for up to 2 years. The study population was treated for analysis as 5 successive 2-year cohorts, and the trend in mortality and the contrast between the first and last cohorts were presented (13).

In Auckland, New Zealand, studies were conducted in 1974 and 1981 in which the survival of MI patients from the date of diagnosis was determined. Survival curves are presented for both cohorts for the year after MI, with numerical results given for the periods up to 28 days, between 28 days and 6 months, and between 6 months and 1 year. These data were then compared between the cohorts identified in the two respective calendar years (14).

The study of Du Pont workers in the U.S. included more than 6000 cases of MI, with short-term mortality recorded from the date of diagnosis. Death within 24 hours (SUD) was presented separately, then included in the events within 30 days of diagnosis, and finally excluded from the period from 1-30 days. Mortality in these time intervals was expressed as average annual rates for the successive 3-year cohorts identified from 1957-1983. Overall trends, the contrasts between the earliest and latest cohorts, were presented (15).

For the population of Worcester, MA, both short- and long-term survival after MI were reported. Cases were identified as of the time of diagnosis, and survival in-hospital and post-discharge to the end of follow-up from 2.5-8.0 years later were determined. For in-hospital survival, the three one-year cohorts of 1975, 1978 and 1981 were compared. For post-hospital survival, each cohort was described by a survival curve carried forward to 1983; all three cohorts could be compared only to the 3-year point in follow up (16).

These brief characterizations of the design of the 9 studies indicate something of their methodologic differences. At a level of greater detail, still further features would be noted as distinguishing one study from another.

Of paramount importance for the present review is to recognize the differences in time reference among these studies. Such differences are crucial in understanding the results which follow, because irrespective of other determinants the apparent survival patterns are influenced strongly by two factors: the state of the disease at the start of observation for each case, and the duration of follow up relative to the initial hours and days of especially high mortality, if these are included in the experience reported. In might therefore be expected that those studies, or specific analyses, which address very short-term survival might show temporal patterns of change which differ importantly from those which exclude it. With this appreciation of the individual studies, their results can now be considered.

**STUDIES OF SURVIVAL AFTER MI:  RESULTS**

The results of these studies are summarized in Table 2.  For each study the time patterns of mortality are denoted either as "CFR" or otherwise to distinguish the shorter- and longer-term observations.  It should be emphasized that "case-fatality rate" (CFR) is used generically here for any of the several constructions of short-term mortality, irrespective of the inclusion of SUD or the first 24-hour period, and whether limited by a fixed interval such as 28 or 30 days or by the date of hospital discharge.  Except for the tendency to restrict "case-fatality" to the hours or days immediately following onset of MI the term does not have consistent usage in this area of study and cannot be interpreted accurately without reference to the survival periods actually studied, as described in Table 1. The longer-range survival is variously denoted in Table 2 in terms more specific to each report.

Short-Term Survival

Patterns of change in short-term survival were reported from 7 of these 9 studies, excluding the HIP and Goteborg populations (Nos. 4 and 6).  In 5 of these studies, decreases in the CFR were demonstrated in one or more of the comparisons made and ranged from 13.9% within 24 hours to 53.0% between 1 and 30 days (both in the Du Pont study) (15).  The decreases were most often to rates between 20 and 30% lower than those of the earliest period of observation.

Not all of these results were wholly consistent even within studies, however.  In Baltimore, the CFR decreased 26.6% for hospitalized patients who were admitted to coronary care units (CCUs) but increased 20.2% for those not in CCUs.  This was in striking contrast to the relative survival in the first year of that study, when rates were the same whether in or out of the CCU (7).  Because CCU care become the predominant form in the later period, the overall result would be a decline in in-hospital mortality for MI patients as a whole in Baltimore.

In Rochester, the CFR between 1 and 30 days decreased by 50% from the first four 5-year cohorts to the last one reported as of 1981.  The extension of this study reported in 1986, however, indicated that mortality in this interval within the acute phase of

**TABLE 1.** Studies of Survival: Summary Description

| No. | Population Studied | Ref. | Year | Calendar Period | Population Size | Age Range | Condition(s) Studied |
|---|---|---|---|---|---|---|---|
| 1. | Baltimore | 7 | 1979 | 1966-67, 1971 | --- | --- | MI |
| 2. | Kaiser-Permanente | 8 | 1979 | 1971-1977 | 430,000 | 35-84 | MI |
| 3. | Rochester (MN) | 9 / 10 | 1981 / 1986 | 1950-1975 / 1950-1982 | 28,000-55,000 | 30+ | MI/SUD |
| 4. | HIP | 11 | 1982 | 1961-1978 | --- | 35-64 | MI |
| 5. | Minneapolis-St. Paul | 12 | 1983 | 1970, 1980 | 1,500,000-2,000,000 | 30-74 | MI |
| 6. | Goteborg | 13 | 1984 | 1968-1977 | --- | < 34-59 | MI |
| 7. | Auckland | 14 | 1984 | 1974, 1981 | 220,000-280,000 | 35-69 | MI (incl. SUD) |
| 8. | Du Pont | 15 | 1985 | 1957-1983 | 88,000-109,000 | 25-65 | MI (incl. SUD) |
| 9. | Worcester (MA) | 16 | 1986 | 1975,1978,1981 | 373,000 | 25+ | MI |

| No. | Number of Cases | Start of Observation | Survival Periods | Trends Examined |
|---|---|---|---|---|
| 1. | 1307 | Hospital admission/ Hospital discharge | In-hospital, with 24-48 hr excl./Post-discharge to 6-10 yrs | Two periods compared |
| 2. | --- | Hospital admission | In hospital | Annual rates over period |
| 3. | 1321/544 1818/694 | Diagnosis | Within 24 hrs/1-30 days/ 5 yrs/31 days - 10 yrs | Consecutive 4-5 yr periods Survival curves to 10 yrs |
| 4. | 436/697 | Post-hospital exam (within 12 mos.) | Exam to 4-5 yrs | Survival curves for 2 cohorts, 1960s v 1970s |
| 5. | 3842/3736 | Hospital admission | In-hospital | Two periods compared |
| 6. | 1322 | Hospital discharge | Post-discharge to 2 yrs | Consecutive 2-yr cohorts |
| 7. | 288 (sample)/ 876 | Diagnosis | Diagnosis to 28 days/28 days to 6 mos/6 most to 1 yr | Consecutive 2-yr cohorts, 1974 v 1981 |
| 8. | 6286 | Diagnosis | Within 24 hrs/within 30 days/1-30 days | Consecutive 3-year cohorts, esp. first v last |
| 9. | 1678 | Diagnosis | In-hospital/Post-discharge to 2.5-8.0 yrs | Three 1-year cohorts for in-hospital survival; survival curves for 3 cohorts all to 1983 |

**TABLE 2:** Studies of Survival: Results and Authors' Interpretations

| No. | Results | Authors' Interpretations |
|---|---|---|
| 1. | -CFR: decreased 26.6% in CCU patients; increased 20.2% in non-CCU patients<br>-Post-discharge survival: unchanged to 5 yrs | -CCU care had impact on mortality by second period studied<br>-Lack of medical care effect on progression of disease or extent of infarct |
| 2. | -CFR: unchanged over period | -Mortality trend in U.S. not due to more effective treatment |
| 3. | -CFR: SUD decreased 40% from peak; 1-30 days CFR decreased 50% (later increased 18.5%, declared 'stable')<br>-Post-30 day survival: unchanged to 8 yrs<br>-Post-exam survival: no important difference in overall mortality | -Only in latest of (original) 5 yr period did change in CFR contribute to change mortality; decreasing CFR with stable later survival does contribute to decrease<br>-Any important medical care contribution to decline in mortality must have been in acute stage |
| 4. | | |
| 5. | -CFR: decreased 29% and 27% in M, F 45-74; increased 26.5%, 32.1% in M, F 35-44 | -No one explanation sufficient for decline in mortality |
| 6. | -Post-discharge survival: decreased "28%" from first to last cohort | -Decrease attributed to increased use of beta-blockers |
| 7. | -CFR, longer-term survival: no significant differences between periods, with or without exclusion of SUD | -No contribution of medical care to decrease in mortality in New Zealand |
| 8. | -CFR: decreased 13.9% within 24 hours; 20.1% within 30 days; 53.0% 1-30 days | -Some contribution of emergency services, hospital treatment for survivors past 24 hrs, to decrease in mortality |
| 9. | -CFR; decreased 21.3%<br>-Post-discharge survival: no change among cohorts to 1 yr; earliest cohort best to 3 yrs | -Improvement in early survival contributed to decrease in mortality; could be due to improved treatment, change in natural history, or prognostic mix of cases |

MI had subsequently increased by 18.5% and then become "stable" (9,10). Thus the CFRs over successive 4- or 5-year periods may fluctuate, and observations based on comparison of only two points or intervals in time may not reflect the true pattern of change over more extended periods. This realization should lead to caution in interpretation of the latter types of comparisons or those in which the contrast of first and last periods of study are emphasized.

The study in Minneapolis-St. Paul indicated an age-sex pattern in changing CFRs. For both men and women decreases in in-hospital death were observed except for patients under 45 years of age, for whom the rates increased. The increase was most dramatic for young women but was based on a relatively low rate in the initial period, 3.4% in 1970 (12).

In two of these studies which included observations of early mortality, the CFR was unchanged over time. This was the case in 8 successive years in the Kaiser-Permanente population of Northern California and between the two calendar years compared, 1974 and 1981, in Auckland (Nos. 2 and 7). In the latter case, this absence of change obtained whether or not SUD was excluded (8, 14).

Longer-Term Survival

Observations of longer-term survival are presented for 6 of the 9 studies, now excluding the Kaiser-Permanente, Minneapolis-St. Paul and Du Point populations (Nos. 2, 5, and 8). These assessments were based on various definitions of the study period: beginning with hospital discharge, the time not otherwise specified, in 3 studies (Nos. 1, 6 and 9); following 28 or 30 days, irrespective of hospital discharge, in 2 studies (Nos. 3 and 7); and following a baseline examination up to several months after hospital discharge, in 1 study (No. 4).

Only one of these 6 studies, that in Goteborg, demonstrated any trend in longer-term mortality after MI (No. 6) (13). The survival curves among three cohorts studied in Worcester in fact indicated that the most favorable experience was in the earliest of the three periods, 1975, v. 1978 or 1981 (No. 9) (16). The decrease in post-discharge survival of MI patients in Goteborg was reported as 28% from the earliest to the latest cohort (although recalculation of this difference based on the smoothed regression curves indicates a decrease of 37.5%) (13). For the remainder of the studies, with follow up over periods from 1 to 8 or 10 years for each of two or more distinct patient cohorts, no trend in survival was found.

The Authors' Interpretations

The authors' interpretations of these varied results recall to mind the several competing or perhaps complementary theories to explain "the decline". In general the results were taken by the authors at face value and interpreted as reflecting the presence or absence of a medical care effect on the changes in CHD mortality occurring more broadly. In the case of an observed decrease in the CFRs, it was most often suggested that improvement in emergency services, CCUs, or hospital treatment more generally was the explanation and that this effect must contribute to the overall decline in CHD mortality. The Rochester group of investigators were more circumspect and simply noted that the magnitude of the decrease and its timing were sufficient to make a true contribution to the subsequent CHD mortality changes observed for the community as a whole. They did not speculate on the basis for the decrease in the CFR in the early 1970s or its lesser increase in the next period of observation (9,10).

Those who observed no change in CFRs, authors of the Kaiser-Permanente and the Auckland study reports (Nos. 2 and 7), concluded that the mortality trends for the U.S. and New Zealand, respectively, could not be explained by more effective hospital treatment or improved medical care more generally (8, 14).

With respect to longer-term survival, the lack of any trend in the majority of studies was accompanied by attributions of no effect on CHD mortality by medical care or restriction of any such effect to the acute phase of treatment for MI. The Baltimore group, who had observed a decrease in CFR associated with CCUs but no longer-term trend, concluded that acute care did have an impact on CHD mortality but that the progression of the underlying pathology or the extent of cardiac damage in the acute phase had not been altered by treatment (7).

The one exceptional finding was that from Goteborg, in which the singular decrease in post-hospital survival was attributed to the very widespread use of beta-blockers which developed over the study period, 1968-1979 (13).

In contrast to the foregoing interpretations, the authors of the reports from both Minneapolis-St. Paul and Worcester suggested that no one explanation was clearly sufficient for the general decline in CHD mortality and that both treatment effects and other influences on the natural history of CHD could be important contributors. By implication, they judged none of the possible explanations to have been excluded by their observations (12, 16).

## CONCLUSIONS

The three questions posed earlier in this review can now be answered as follows:

1. Trends have been demonstrated in survival after MI in several but not all studies. In general a decrease of 20 - 30% in early mortality was observed, while after the first days or weeks no change in survival occurred.

2. Exceptions must be noted for younger subjects or for certain whole study populations where different results were obtained. To judge how closely consistent the results of the remaining studies are would require much more detailed consideration of diagnostic criteria and other aspects of study design than is possible here.

3. Interpretations by the investigators in this area are varied. A sense of the conclusions common to several of the reports is that medical care, in the acute phase of MI, may well have altered the early mortality from MI in several populations and that this has likely contributed to the broader trends in CHD mortality. Past the acute phase, however, little impact of treatment on mortality is evident; Goteborg is an apparent exception. Other influences on the natural history of CHD have not been excluded as contributory to the trends in overall CHD mortality.

It may be useful in closing to note some of the further questions, raised by the answers above, which are especially pertinent to these deliberations:

1. If we accept that the proportion of cases of MI surviving the acute phase is changing, how might the composition of this population be changing as well? Are the clinical profiles, especially indicators of prognosis, changing in ways which should influence management in the short term or later? Goldberg and others address this question in two reports reviewed here which suggest the importance of this question (7, 16).

2. If late survival has not in general been altered, even where acute-phase mortality has decreased, what implications are raised for further development of therapy? The Goteborg example is difficult to replicate in settings where the actual treatment of the target population is less well documented; the need is suggested for detailed studies of actual post-MI treatment and other factors potentially influencing prognosis in this late phase in the progression of CHD.

3. What might we predict as future trends in early and late mortality among patients with MI? The determinants of future trends may well include, on present evidence, innovations in acute-phase treatment. Discovery why those developments in the past do not appear to have had an impact in the post-hospital phase would be important and may suggest ways in which existing measures can be made more effective. Further study of the post-hospital course and its possible pre- and in-hospital predictors could contribute to such an understanding.

Finally, it remains to observe that the natural history of CHD, including its modification by treatment, continues to elude explanation in many fundamental ways. From an epidemiologic perspective, all of the questions just posed address only one aspect of a much more complex problem: This is to know how the population is changing from which the cases of MI arise, how and why those who experience MI or other clinically manifest CHD are changing as a subset of that population, and how the component causes that have been identified can be further modified by practical preventive measures as well as by treatment of recognized diseases.

The changing patterns in the epidemiology of CHD have brought the realization that this natural history is more dynamic and more diverse in different population settings than was often appreciated in the past. This variation in natural history in time and place presents many challenges. It also offers opportunities to be exploited for the benefit of both the population at large and, in particular, those who continue to experience MI.

**REFERENCES**
1. Havlik, R.J., Feinleib, M. Eds. Proceedings of the Conference on the Decline in Coronary Heart Disease Mortality, US Dept HEW, PHS, NIH, NIH Publ. No. 79-1610, 1979.
2. Stallones, R.A. Sci. Am. 243: 53-59, 1980.
3. Ueshima, H., Cooper, R., Stamler, J., et al. J. Chron. Dis. 37: 425-439, 1984.
4. Davis, W.B., Hayes, C.G., Knowles, M., et al. Am. J. Epidemiol. 122: 657-672, 1985.
5. Pisa, Z., Uemura, K. Trends of mortality from ischaemic heart disease and other cardiovascular diseases in 27 countries, 1968-1977. World Hlth Stat. Q. 35: 11-47, 1982.
6. Thom, T.J., Epstein, F.H., Feldman, J.J., Leaverton, P.E. Int. J. Epidemiol. 14: 510-520, 1985.
7. Goldberg, R., Szklo, M., Tonascia, J.A., Kennedy, H.L. Johns Hopkins Med. J. 144: 73-80, 1979.
8. Friedman, G.D. In: Proceedings of the Conference on the Decline in Coronary Heart Disease Mortality (Eds. R.J. Havlik & M. Feinleib), US Dept HEW, PHS, NIH, NIH Publ. No. 79-1610, 1979.
9. Elveback, L.R., Connolly, D.C., Kurland, L.T. Mayo Clin. Proc. 56: 665-672, 1981.
10. Elveback, L.R., Connolly, D.C., Melton III, L.J. Mayo Clin. Proc. 61: 896-900, 1986.
11. Weinblatt, E., Goldberg, J.D., Ruberman, W., et al. JAMA 247: 1576-1581, 1982.
12. Gillum, R.F., Folsom, A., Luepker, R.V., et al. N. Engl. J. Med. 309: 1353-1358, 1983.
13. Aberg, A., Bergstrand, R., Johansson, S., et al. Br. Heart J. 51: 346-351, 1984.
14. Stewart, A.W., Fraser, G.E., Beaglehole, R., Sharpe, D.N. Lancet 444-446, 1984.
15. Pell, S., Fayerweather, W.E. N. Engl. J. Med. 312: 1005-1010, 1985.
16. Goldberg, R.J., Gore, J.M., Alpert, J.S., Dalen, J.E. JAMA 255: 2774-2779, 1986.

# 3

## TRENDS IN PRE-HOSPITAL MORTALITY

C. T. Kappagoda

Department of Medicine, University of Alberta Hospitals, Edmonton, Alberta, Canada T6G 2R7

### INTRODUCTION

Myocardial infarction is a clinical syndrome in which there is a variable delay between the onset of symptoms and entry into hospital or even summoning of medical assistance. Indeed many episodes of myocardial infarction go undetected clinically (1). Due to the particular temporal relationship between the onset of symptoms and the occurence of events that appear in conventional analyses of prognosis, it is essential to distinguish between the experience reported from hospitals and that reported from community surveys. An accurate estimate of the prognosis could be obtained only on the basis of the overall incidence of the condition in the community.

The prognosis that is considered during the course of conventional hospital practice would refer either to a subset of patients who have been admitted to the hospital or only to a group of patients who have survived the period of hospitalization. Thus community surveys such as those reported from Framingham (2) and Rochester (3) present a view of the problem which differs from that depicted in reports from tertiary care institutions (4). The latter is likely to be distorted further by the propensity for centers of excellence to attract patients with major clinical problems.

### HISTORICAL PERSPECTIVES

In the 1950's several reports appeared in the literature defining the so-called primary mortality from myocardial infarction. In most instances this term represented the mortality within the first 4 weeks after the initial diagnosis. In others it was taken to indicate the in-hospital mortality. Usually the diagnosis was based upon 1) a history of pain in the chest, 2) electrocardiographic changes of myocardial infarction, 3) a leukocytosis, and 4) fever.

Biorck et al. in 1957 (5) reported the experience from Malmo in Sweden covering a period from 1935 to 1954. They found that out of a total of 1,530 patients admitted to the department of medicine with their first episode of infarction, 556 (36.3%) died during their stay in hospital and 500 (32.7%) did so within 4 weeks of admission. The data from other Scandinavian centers during this period were similar (5,6,7). The majority of North American and European centers reported statistics for this period to indicate that approximately one-third of such patients died during this initial 6-8 week period (8-11).

However, it must be emphasized that these studies were all retrospective in nature and based upon patients admitted to hospital with a myocardial infarction. The clinical data were analyzed subsequently, and only those patients deemed not to have sustained a previous infarct were retained for analysis. It is unlikely that such a claim could have been substantitaed with the diagnostic tools available at the time, particularly in view of subsequent findings from Framingham (12) and the New York Health Insurance Plan (13), which indicated that a substantial proportion of infarcts remained undetected clinically during the acute phase. Nevertheless, Helander and Levander in 1959 (6) and Biorck et al. in 1957 (5) made a specific attempt to include only those patients with their first episode of infarction, and both groups reported very similar mortality values of 36.3% and 32%, respectively, over the initial 6-8 weeks.

In contrast, two investigations reported from the United States indicated a significantly better prognosis in these patients. Cole et al. in 1954 (14) reported a mortality of 23% during the first 2 months after infarction in a study which covered the period from 1932 to 1942, and Juergens et al. in 1960 (15) reported a primary mortality of 16% over a period of 17 years between 1934 and 1951. These apparent differences between the European and American data merit further scrutiny. One answer to the problem could be obtained from the 25-year follow up of 200 patients with myocardial infarction reported by Richards et al. in 1956 (16). The immediate (4 week) mortality in their study was 19%. They pointed out that "the fact that the series has been obtained from a consultation practice (White's) must be taken into consideration in order to properly evaluate the 'immediate mortality.' Many patients had already survived the acute period before they came under observation. On the other hand, it should be recognized that consultation in many instances was prompted by a situation more serious than usual, thus weighing the series toward the more severe cases." However, sudden death during the early phases of myocardial infarction is not always preceded by a clinical syndrome suggesting a potentially life-threatening situation (see below). Thus, one could speculate that the relatively low mortality reported from some of the more prestigious institutions in the United States reflected an inadvertent selection of patients.

Such a point of view is supported by the findings of the Health Insurance Plan of Greater New York reported more than a decade later (13). This particular investigation was based upon a follow up of new cases of myocardial infarction over a 4-year period which commenced on November 1, 1961. Eight hundred and eighty-one patients who suffered a first episode of infarction were identified. Of these, 217 patients died without reaching hospital. In contrast, 601 patients were hospitalized for a first myocardial infarction and, of these, 17% died within the first month. This figure is comparable with the data reported by Cole et al. in 1954 (14), Juergens et al. in 1960 (15), and Richards et al. in 1956 (16). However, out of the original group of 881 patients, 271 died during the first 24 hours (the majority of them before reaching hospital).

In summary, it could be concluded that up to 1950 the overall mortality rate reported in patients admitted to hospital following an initial infarction was approximately 20% in North American centers.

In the 1960s the advent of coronary care units caused major changes in the manner in which patients were managed after a myocardial infarction, particularly with respect to the treatment of ventricular arrhythmias. In order to appreciate the impact of these changes, they have to be viewed against one other factor, namely, the early mortality after infarction.

In Belfast, McNeilly and Pemberton in 1968 (17) conducted a retrospective analysis of approximately 1,000 patients whose cause of death had been stated as myocardial infarction. Of these patients, 40% had died within 1 hour after the onset of symptoms. A further 15% died over the next 3 hours. Sixty percent of the deaths had occurred with 12 hours. Although this study was based primarily upon the analysis of death certificates, it was supported also by very painstaking inquiries from relatives (Fig. 1).

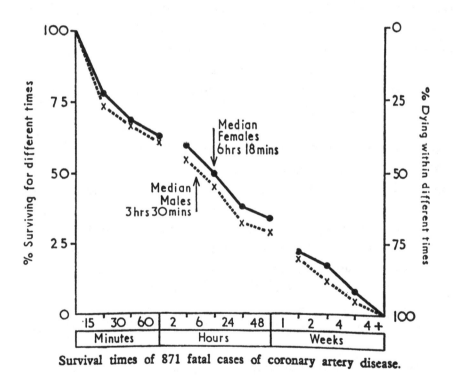

Survival times of 871 fatal cases of coronary artery disease.

**FIGURE 1.** Survival after the onset of symptoms in patients dying following myocardial infarction. The data were based upon a group of 871 patients whose cause of death had been certified as myocardial infarction. It is seen that approximately 40% of the deaths occurred during the first hour. It was found that in the 602 patients in whom the information was available the median interval from the onset of symptoms to the time a doctor was sent for was approximately 70 minutes. [Reproduced by permission from the editor, Br. Med. J. McNeilly and Pemberton (1968).]

In general, these findings support the basic position of the New York Health Insurance Plan study (13), which suggested that nearly 70% of deaths after a first infarction occurred within the first 24 hours.

The impact of coronary care units on the mortality from myocardial infarction has to be viewed against this background. Levenstein in 1976 (18) reviewed the literature over a 15-year period and described the evolution of these units in North America, the United Kingdom and Australia. He showed that in 17 reports which appeared over a 6-year period from 1965, the average mortality was 17.6% (range 14-22%) (5 of these reports quoted mortality rates for control populations which ranged from 27 to 35%). From these findings it was difficult to conclude with any certainty that coronary care units of the sort operational in the late 1960s had any significant impact on the mortality in patients admitted to hospital with myocardial infarcts. Nevertheless, Levenstein concluded that "although statisticians may argue, cardiologists were satisfied with the efficiency of the intensive coronary care unit."

These somewhat disappointing results over the period reviewed by Levenstein (18) could be attributed to the distribution of the deaths with respect to the onset of symptoms leading to myocardial infarction. Peel et al. in 1962 (19), Norris et al. in 1969 (20), and Honey and Truelove in 1957 (21) have shown that the majority of deaths occurred within the first 24 hours spent in hospital, provided the patients were admitted within the first 6 hours of the illness (Fig. 2). These studies, taken in conjunction with the epidemiological investigations of McNeilly and Pemberton in 1970 (17) and Weinblatt et al. in 1968 (13) show that the majority of deaths following infarction occurred during the first few hours after onset of the symptoms. Thus, coronary care units were likely to benefit patients who sought hospitalization early in the course of their illness.

Stern in 1979 (22), in a critical analysis of the factors which influenced the overall statistics which emanated from coronary care units, highlighted some of the practical difficulties involved in assessing the data. He emphasized two important points which bedevil this problem.

1.  Most of the evidence cited to prove that coronary care units lower the hospital fatality due to myocardial infarction was based upon historical rather than concurrent controls.

2.  Only two randomized clinical trials, both in England, have been done (23,24,25), neither of which showed an advantage for coronary care units.

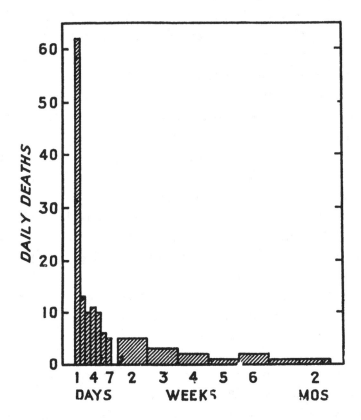

**FIGURE 2.** Survival of patients admitted to hospital with an acute myocardial infarction. The majority of these deaths occurred during the first 24 hr. The data were obtained during a period when coronary care units were not available and based upon an analysis of 543 admissions to hospital. [Reproduced with permission from Honey and Truelove (1957).]

Nevertheless, Stern (22) concluded that coronary care units probably contributed to the overall decline in the mortality from

ischemic heart disease observed in the United States. This
conclusion was based principally on the contention that the decline
in the mortality from ischemic heart disease observed in the late
1960s and early 1970s in the United States could not be explained by
changes in the risk-factor profile of the population of the United
States during that period. Equally, it could not be explained by the
advent of coronary bypass surgery which in numerical terms alone
would not have made a significant impact on the problem during the
period under review.

## DEVELOPMENT OF MOBILE CORONARY CARE UNITS

Once it was recognized generally that the majority of the early
deaths due to infarction occurred during the first few hours after
the onset of symptoms, the concept of mobile coronary care was born.
Pantridge and his colleagues (26) in 1972 in Belfast, in particular,
argued that if the patients could be reached within the first hour,
it would be possible to take lifesaving measures and thereby
influence the mortality trends favorably.

Pantridge and Adgey (26) reported their initial experience
between 1966 and 1969 with such a mobile unit. During this period
the mobile unit made 2,753 calls (Table 1). Of these, 43% were for
patients who subsequently developed unequivocal evidence of
infarction. A further 33% had acute coronary insufficiency. Of the
patients who had sustained an infarction, approximately 25% came
under care within 1 hour, 52% within 2 hours, and 75% within 4 hours
of the onset of symptoms. The patients seen within 1 hour had a
variety of disturbances which merited therapy before they were deemed
fit to be moved to hospital. During this same period, 193 patients
required resuscitation outside the hospital, and it was suggested
that this group represented the potential salvage of patients with
this mode of management.

Following these reports, mobile coronary care teams were created
in Great Britain, the United States, and Europe (27,28,29). Many of
these groups have reported results in recent years, and these are too
numerous to review in detail here.

**TABLE 1.** Incidence of Dysrhythmias Among 284 Patients Seen Within the First Hour by a Mobile Coronary Care Team

|  | No. of Patients Within First Hour | Total No. of Patients |
| --- | --- | --- |
| Bradyarrhythmia | 88 (31%) | 124 (44%) |
| Ventricular ectopics | 70 (24.6%) | 163 (57.4%) |
| Ventricular tachycardia | 10 (3.5%) | 87 (30.6%) |
| Ventricular fibrillation | 28 (9.9%) | 54 (19%) |
| Atrial fibrillation | 11 (3.9%) | 26 (9.1%) |
| Supraventricular tachycardia | 1 (0.35%) | 11 (3.9%) |

Source:  From Pantridge and Adgey, 1972 (26)

It must be emphasized that these studies, although excellent in many respects, did not take the form of conventional clinical trials. In order to rectify this obvious anomaly Hamptom and his colleagues in Nottingham, England, undertook a randomized clinical trial to assess the efficacy of a mobile coronary care unit (MCCU) (30).  Over a 15-month period, a total of 6,223 calls for emergency ambulances were considered for the study.  Of these, 1,664 patients were allocated to the MCCU while 1,676 were allocated to the routine ambulance.  In these groups, the prehospital mortality in patients with heart attacks was 45 and 47% respectively.  None of the patients who required resuscitation survived long enough to leave hospital. These findings ran against the prevailing trends in coronary care.

One factor which drew a great deal of the criticism for this report was the outcome in patients in whom resuscitation was attempted.  The procedure was attempted in 32 patients, and only 2 were alive at the time of admission to hospital.  The latter result was used to cast aspersions on the technical competence of the staff of the MCCU (31).  While this claim remains speculative, there were two other issues which merited scrutiny.

The first was that the sample sizes were very small (only 133 patients with confirmed myocardial infarctions were randomized); second, approximately 50% of the patients randomized in the study were seen by the ambulance staff within 1/2 hour of the onset of symptoms, while 70% were seen within 1 hour.  There is little one can add about the former. The latter has an important bearing upon the overall mortality from myocardial infarction, particularly in terms of the possibility of a successful outcome from an attempted resuscitation.

As indicated previously, many investigations have confirmed that the majority of the <u>deaths</u> following an infarction occurred within the first hour (27,32). The effect of prompt intervention in such patients was investigated by Eisenberg et al. in 1979 (33) who reported their experience with a group of patients who developed an episode of cardiac arrest outside the hospital: 38-40% of those who received cardiopulmonary resuscitation (CPR) within 4 minutes and definitive treatment within 9 minutes recovered and were discharged from hospital. They showed also that the percentage of patients discharged from hospital was inversely proportional to the delay in initiating CPR and in providing definite coronary care. These findings could explain the disappointing result in the report by Hampton and Nicholas in 1978 (30).

Thus, there appears to be ample justification for the belief that the rapid provision of coronary care which takes the form of MCCU and public participation in a CPR program could reduce the hospital mortality in patients (34).

The justification for this claim is not based upon controlled clinical trials but on comparisons with historical controls (27) which show a significant reduction in community mortality rate attributable to myocardial infarction during a preceding period. This approach has many pitfalls, particularly when it is viewed against a background of diminishing trends in mortality from myocardial infarction (22). Another approach to the provision of evidence in support of the claim that these mobile units influence overall mortality stems from mortality statistics in groups of users and nonusers of the mobile coronary care system. The dangers of this approach are indicated in the data reported by Lewis et al. in 1982 (35). Table 2, derived from their report, shows the distribution of the characteristics of the patients admitted to the hospital.

As the authors themselves point out, it is difficult to draw any definite conclusion from these findings. Clearly, the two populations are not similar to one another, and there are several possible explanations for this. Patients could have perceived correctly the severity of their illness and sought the help of the mobile coronary care unit. Alternatively, many of the more seriously ill patients could have died before summoning help and reaching the hospital. The authors believed that ignorance about the existence of the service was not a factor and that the decision made by the patients to (or not to) activate the mobile coronary care unit was a clinically appropriate one. The truth is clearly to be found somewhere between these extremes.

**TABLE 2.** Distribution of Selected Characteristics of Patients Who Activated a Mobile Coronary Care System[a]

| Characteristics[b] | Users | Nonusers |
|---|---|---|
| N | 274 | 270 |
| Age | 62.6 + 12 | 61.3 + 11 |
| Male (%) | 69 | 77 |
| Time onset Sx to Rx[c] | 45 min | 252 min |
|   With incapacitating Sx (%) | 55 | 37 |
|   With transmural MI %) | 71 | 71 |
|   With Peak SGOT 100 IU/ml (%) | 55 | 37 |
|   With serious complications(%) | 53 | 16 |
| Hospital mortality rate | 16.7% | 1.5% |

[a]Explanatory note: It appears that the nonusers had fewer symptoms, smaller infarcts, and fewer complications than the users. The mortality rate in hospital was lower also. The authors suggested that the nonusers made the clinically appropriate decision in delaying the call to the mobile unit.

[b]Cardiac arrest, pulmonary edema, shock, or hypotension-bradycardia syndrome (includes prehospital and new hospital events). Significant at $p < 0.05$ (users versus nonusers).

[c]Rx, arrival of MCCU or arrival at hospital emergency room for nonusers; Sx, symptoms

## THE NATURE OF SUDDEN DEATH

In attempting to establish the impact of mobile coronary care units on the hospital mortality in patients with infarction, it is important to consider the nature of sudden cardiac death a little further.

Community studies such as those undertaken at Framingham (36) and Albany (37) show that approximately 40% of sudden deaths (less than one hour after the onset of symptoms) occurred in men with no prior evidence of coronary artery disease while nearly 60% of all sudden deaths occurred in apparently asymptomatic men. The incidence of sudden death in Framingham was 1.5, 3.6 and 3.2/1000/year for men aged 45-54, 55-64 and 65-74 years respectively.

An episode of cardiac arrest, when it occurs in patients with infarction (i.e., secondary ventricular fibrillation) is a significant independent predictor of subsequent mortality (38). When such an episode complicates an infarction, a high proportion of the patients die in hospital (e.g. 55% in the study reported by Conley et al. (38) in 1977), and the subsequent course of the patient appears to depend on the severity of the infarct. In contrast, when ventricular fibrillation occurs in patients without evidence of infarction (i.e. primary ventricular fibrillation), the outcome is quite different. For instance, Lawrie et al. in 1968 (39) reported a hospital mortality of only 17% for such patients in contrast to 72% for patients with secondary ventricular fibrillation. These considerations carry certain implications for the results in patients resuscitated by a mobile coronary care team. One of the largest series reported is that from the Harbor View Medical Center in Seattle (28). Over a 4-year period, their team resuscitated 234 patients (245 episodes) who were subsequently discharged from hospital. This number represented 11% of attempts in the first 2 years and 23% of attempts in the second 2 years.

During the subsequent follow up period (average 437 days), 72 patients died while 11 were resuscitated a second time, making a total of 83 events. Of 39 instances where ventricular fibrillation was associated with electrocardiographic evidence of transmural infarction (Q waves), 5 deaths occurred, and in the 200 episodes where no such evidence was available, 70 deaths and/or recurrences occurred. Further, taking the enzymatic evidence for infarction alone, 20% of patients with such evidence were dead after 1 year and 28% after 2 years. The corresponding values for patients without enzymatic evidence of necrosis were 32 and 47% respectively. It is also of interest to note that 30 patients in this series had recurrent episodes of ventricular fibrillation at an average time of 28 weeks after the first episode (median, 17 weeks).

Thus, the patients resuscitated by mobile coronary care teams do not seem to be a homogeneous group. Ventricular fibrillation that occurs secondary to a myocardial infarction probably represents a specific clinical entity with a relatively favorable long-term prognosis when compared with ventricular fibrillation which occurs as a primary event. It appears that the latter phenomenon could be reversed with relative ease but carries a significant predisposition for recurrence. This possibility has to be borne in mind when evaluating the potential impact of mobile coronary care units on the community mortality and the hospital mortality from myocardial infarction.

Norris and Sammel in 1980 (4) examined the changing patterns in the hospital mortality in patients under 70 years of age. They reported that 14% of patients admitted to the Coronary Care Unit of the Green Lane Hospital, Auckland, New Zealand, died during their stay at the hospital. This unit is supplemented by the services of an ambulance based life support system and the period under review was from July, 1977, to June, 1979. Table 3 shows the major causes of death in these patients contrasted with the experience ten years earlier. As the investigators indicate, the main changes in the causes of death have been in the consequences of arrhythmias. With the decline in arrhythmia related deaths, the mechanical consequences of cardiac failure and rupture have acquired greater importance as modes of death in hospital.

These findings which can be corroborated from reports from several other centers support the proposition that in circumstances where coronary care units can be supplemented by a mobile coronary care facility, mortality in hospital approaching 10-12% can be anticipated in patients under the age of 70 years.

In this context it is of interest to consider the workers of E.I. duPont Nemours Company of Wilmington (40). This analysis was based upon a sample of approximately 100,000 employees. The data was collected between 1957 and 1983. It was observed that the incidence

**TABLE 3.** Mode of Dying of Hospitalized Patients Treated Before the Introduction of a Coronary Care Unit (1 yr, 1966-1967) Compared With Those Treated in a Coronary Care Unit (2 yr, 1977-1979)

| | Number of Patients (%) | | | |
|---|---|---|---|---|
| Mode of Dying | 1966 - 1967 | | 1977 - 1979 | |
| Arrhythmias | 105 | (52) | 10 | (12) |
| Cardiogenic shock | 54 | (27) | 34 | (41) |
| Cardiac failure | 29 | (14) | 17 | (21) |
| Arrhythmia causing cardiac failure | 3 | (1.5) | 0 | (0) |
| Cardiac rupture | 3 | (1.5) | 8 + 6? | (10 + 7)? |
| Pulmonary embolus | 2 | (1) | 1 | (1) |
| Other causes | 6 | (3) | 7 | (8) |
| Total deaths | 202 | (100) | 83 | (100) |
| Total patients | 757 | | 574 | |
| Percent mortality | 26 | | 14 | |

Source: Reproduced by permission from Norris and Sammel (4)

of myocardial infarction declined during this period. In addition, the 24 hour mortality after the onset of infarction declined from 25.5% in 1957-1959 to 21.6% in 1981-1983, and the 30 day mortality declined from 30.4% to 24.3% during the same period. The researchers speculated that this decline may be due in part to the advances of medical care during this period of time, not the least of which is the provision of effective care early in the course of a myocardial infarction.

**REFERENCES**
1. Bayliss, R.I.S. Br. Med. J. 290: 1093-1094, 1985.
2. Dawber, T.R. The Framingham Study. The epidemiology of atherosclerotic disease. Cambridge, Harvary University Press, 1980.
3. Elveback, L.R. Coronary heart disease in Rochester, Minnesota (1950-1975); incidence and survivorship. In: Havlick, R.S., Feinleib, M. (Eds). Proceedings of the conference on the decline in Coronary Heart Disease Mortality. Washington, D.C., Government Printing Office, p. 116-118, 1979.
4. Norris, R.M., Sammel, N.L. Prog. Cardiovasc. Dis. 23: 129-140, 1980.
5. Biorck, G., Blomqvist, G., Sievers, J. Acta Med. Scand. 159: 253-274, 1957.
6. Helander, S., Levander, M. Acta Med. Scand. 163: 289-304, 1959.

7. Myocardial infarction: an epidemiologic and prognostic study of patients from five departments of internal medicine in Oslo 1935-1949. Acta Med. Scand. (Suppl. 315): 1956.

8. Katz, L. N., Mills, G.Y., Cisneros, F. Arch. intern. Med. 84: 305-320, 1941.

9. Master, A.M., Jaffe, H.L., Dack, S. Am. Heart J. 12: 549-562, 1936.

10. Bland, E.F., White P.D. JAMA 117: 1171-1173, 1941.

11. Gillman, Von H. Cardiologica 27: 235-248, 19855.

12. Kannel, W.B. Am. J. Cardiol. 37: 269-282, 1976.

13. Weinblatt, E., Shapiro, S., Frank, C.W., Sager, R.V. Am. J. Public Health 58: 1329-1347, 1968.

14. Cole, D.E., Singian, E.B., Katz, L.N Circulation 9: 321-334, 1954.

15. Juergens, J.L., Edwards, J.E., Achor, R.W., Burchell, H.B. Arch. Intern. Med. 105: 444-450, 1960.

16. Richards, D.W., Bland, E.F., White, P.D. J. Chron. Dis. 4: 415-422, 1956.

17. McNeilly, R.H., Pemberton, J. Br. Med. J. 3: 139-142, 1968.

18. Levenstein, J.H. S. Afr. Med. J. 50: 918-926, 1976.

19. Peel, A.A., Semple, T., Wang, I., et al. Br. Heart J. 24: 745-760, 1962.

20. Norris, R.M., Caughey, D.E., Deeming, L.W., t al. Lancet 2: 485-487, 1969.

21. Honey, G.E., Truelove, S.C. Lancet 1: 1155-1161, 1957.

22. Stern, M.P. Ann. Intern. Med. 91: 630-640, 1979.

23. Mather, H.G., Pearson, N.G., Read, K.L.Q., et al. Br. Med. J. 3: 334-338, 1971.

24. Mather, H.G., Morgan, D.C., Pearson, N.G., et al. Br. Med. J. 1: 925-929, 1976.

25. Hill, J.D., Hampton J.R., Mitchell, J.R. Lancet 1: 837-841, 1978.

26. Pantridge, J.F., Adgey, A.A. The prehospital phase of acute myocardial infarction. In Textbook of Coronary Care, L.E. Meltzer and A.J. Dunning (eds.). The Charles Press, Philadelphia, p. 95-106, 1972.

27. Crampton, R.S., Aldrich, R.F., Gascho, J.A., et al. Am. J. Med. 54: 151-165, 1975.

28. Cobb, L.A., Baum, R.S., Alvarez, H., Schaffer, W.A. Circulation 51/52, III: 223-235, 1976.

29. Siltanen, P. Sundberg, S., Hytonen, I. Acta. Med. Scand. 205: 195-200, 1979.

30. Hampton, J.R., Nicholas, C. Br. Med. J. 1: 1118-1121, 1978.

31. Adgey, A.A. Am. Heart J. 100: 408, 1980.

32. Colling, A., Dellipiani, A.W., Donaldson, R.J., MacCormack, P. Br. Med. J. 2: 1169-1172, 1976.

33. Eisenberg, M.S., Bergner, L., Hallstrom, A. JAMA 241: 1905-1907, 1979.

34. Thompson, R.G., Hallstrom, A.P., Cobb, L.A. Ann. Intern. Med. 90: 737-740, 1979.

35. Lewis, R.P., Lanese, R.R., Stang, J.M., et al. Am. Heart J. 103: 123-130, 1982.

36. Kannel, W.B., Feinlab, M. Am. J. Cardiol. 29: 154-163, 1972.

37. Kuller, L.H., Cooper, M., Perper, J., Fisher R.   Bull. N.Y. Acad. Med.  49: 532-543, 1973.
38. Conley, M.J., McNeer, J.F., Lee, K.L., Wagner, G.S.   Am. J. Cardiol. 39: 7-12, 1977.
39. Lawrie, D.M., Higgins, M.R., Godman, M.J., et al.   Lancet 2: 523-528, 1968.
40. Peel, S., Fayerweather W.E.   N. Engl. J. Med.  312: 1005-1011, 1985.

# 4

## HOSPITAL AND POST-HOSPITAL MORTALITY AFTER MYOCARDIAL INFARCTION

Robin M. Norris

Coronary-Care Unit, Green Lane Hospital, Auckland, New Zealand

### INTRODUCTION

Mortality from coronary heart disease is on the wane in many countries. Fig. 1 shows age-standardized death rates obtained from death certificates from 1955 to 1983 in non-Maori men and women in New Zealand. A gradual decline in mortality of the order of 20% has occurred in both sexes and in all age groups since 1968. What is the cause of this decline?

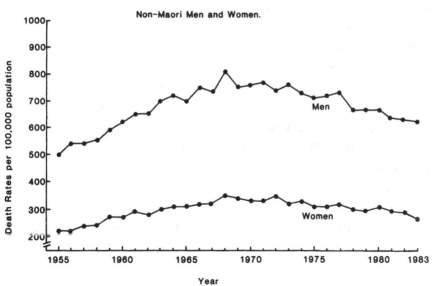

**FIGURE 1.** Age standardized death rates for New Zealand non-Maori men and women 1955-82. (Reproduced with permission from R. Beaglehole and colleagues.)

A number of reasons have been suggested and the chief argument lies between those who believe that deaths from coronary disease have declined because of primary prevention through better diet, more exercise and less smoking in at-risk groups, and those who believe that the decline is due to medical interventions such as coronary care units, coronary artery surgery and beta blocking drugs. My own belief is that causes of the decline are multifactorial and that better treatment of patients with myocardial infarction in hospital has contributed to a large degree to this decline in mortality rate.

Before discussing patterns of change in hospital mortality from acute myocardial infarction it is necessary to stress the one prognostic factor which is unlikely to change, which is the age of the patient. Virtually every study on hospital mortality has shown that mortality increases with age, so that age must always be considered as a potentially confounding variable when one compares the results of different studies. Data discussed in this paper referring to total hospital mortality will refer mainly to patients under 70 years of age and data on the relationship to left ventricular function and coronary anatomy to prognosis will refer only to patients under 60 years of age.

## IMPACT OF HOSPITAL CARE

Hospital mortality from acute myocardial infarction is declining. The continuous line of Fig. 2, which summarizes 18 years of experience in Auckland hospitals, shows a decline in mortality rate following introduction of the first coronary care unit in 1967 and a continuing slower decline over the years since then. Data supporting the 3 earlier points on this graph have been published (1-3), while the 1982 data point refers to experience during the course of a clinical trial (4) conducted between 1981 and 1984 in which the mortality of all patients with verified infarction was documented whether they had been admitted to the clinical trial or not.

Is this decline in mortality due to better hospital treatment or to a decline in severity of the underlying atherosclerotic disease? We showed evidence in 1969 (2) that introduction of

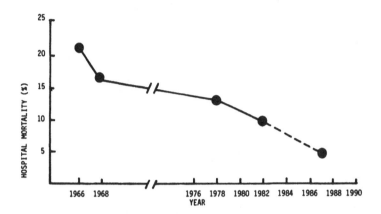

**FIGURE 2.** Hospital mortality from acute myocardial infarction for patients under 70 years of age in Auckland since 1966. Data points until 1982 are based on published surveys (see text for details); the 1987 point is an estimate based on our own experience and that of others (summarized in Figure 4) of the results of thrombolytic trials.

Coronary Care Units had reduced mortality rates during the 1960's, and although this conclusion has been disputed by some, it has been accepted by most authors and by the great majority of cardiologists. Reasons for the continuing decline in mortality during the 1970's are more controversial. It is my belief that improved management, particularly early treatment for shock, cardiac failure and arrhythmias, is the major cause of this slow decline. In Auckland, where admission of patients to a given hospital is determined almost entirely by their zone of residence, there was no change in numbers of patients admitted to our Coronary Care Unit between 1974 and 1983 (Fig. 3).

Recently, Fraser et al (manuscript in preparation) have reviewed 400 x-rays taken after admission to hospital on patients

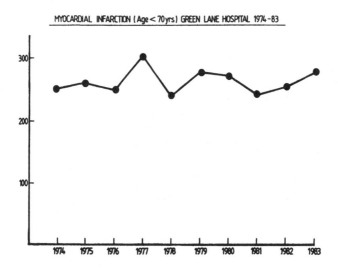

MYOCARDIAL INFARCTION (Age < 70yrs) GREEN LANE HOSPITAL 1974-83

**FIGURE 3.** Numbers of patients admitted to the coronary-care unit of a general hospital from a defined admitting area 1974-83.

with myocardial infarction during 1981 - 1982. The proportions of patients showing cardiac enlargement, venous congestion or pulmonary oedema in these x-rays differed very little in 1981 - 1982 from the proportions in 1966 - 1967 (1). We found in the earlier study that cardiac enlargement and radiological evidence of pulmonary congestion or oedema were the main factors apart from age which determined prognosis, and this finding has been confirmed in subsequent studies. Thus it did not appear that the prognostic index for these patients had changed greatly between 1966 and 1981. Therefore the greater part of the decline in mortality rate was more likely to have been due to better medical management than to admission to hospital of less seriously ill patients.

What of hospital mortality during the 1980's? Now for the first time we have methods of treatment for the myocardial infarct itself rather than for its complications; first, by a reduction of myocardial oxygen demand using intravenous beta blockers, and second (and more important) by reperfusion using thrombolytic drugs or angioplasty. The ISIS Trial (5) showed a 15% reduction in mortality rate (from 4.6% to 3.9%) from intravenous atenolol given within 12 hours of onset of infarction. However, if intravenous beta blockers were to be used routinely, the expected reduction in mortality rate would be less than 15% because the most seriously ill patients have contraindications to administration of beta blocker. Extrapolating from our own experience (4), we found a 5.4% hospital mortality for the 70% of patients who had no contraindications to beta blockers and a 21% mortality for the 30% who did have contraindications, giving a total mortality rate of 10.1%. The routine use of beta blockers in patients who did not have contraindications would be expected to cause a 15% reduction in mortality from 5.4% (i.e. to 4.6%).

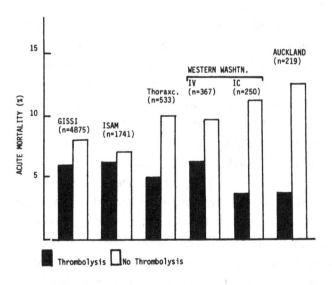

**FIGURE 4.** Reduction in hospital mortality from acute myocardial infarction which has been shown in trials of thrombolytic therapy. Hospital mortality of treated patients is 5% on average. For discussion see text.

However, the reduction in mortality for all patients would be only .6% (from 10.1% to 9.5%). Thus the benefit to be expected in terms of reduction of hospital mortality from acute myocardial infarction by the use of beta blockers is modest.

More promising in terms of the reduction in mortality appears to be the use of thrombolysis by pharmacological agents such as streptokinase or tissue plasminogen activator, or mechanically by means of percutaneous transluminal coronary angioplasty. Fig. 4 summarizes the results of six trials of thrombolysis (6-11). Only the results of trials which involved more than 200 patients are shown in this figure; six of the seven (6-11) were randomized controlled trials and all used streptokinase which was given intravenously in four trials (6,7,9,11) and by the intracoronary route in one (10). One trial used intracoronary and intravenous streptokinase and angioplasty in the treated patients (8). The striking finding from these trials is that for treated patients under 70 years of age hospital mortality did not exceed 6%, and it was 6% also in two of the trials which enrolled patients up to 75 years of age (7,9).

Not only does thrombolysis reduce mortality rate, but we believe that it also improves left ventricular function for surviving patients. In the Auckland study (11) 98% of surviving patients had coronary arteriography and left ventriculography at three weeks after infarction. Ejection fraction was significantly higher in patients who had had streptokinase than in control patients (59 $\pm$ 1% [SEM] v 53 $\pm$ 2%; p $<$ 0.005), end-systolic volume was lower (55 $\pm$ 3 ml v 73 $\pm$ 5 ml; p $<$ 0.005) and the contractility score assessed from visual inspection of biplane ventriculograms was better in treated patients (2.9 $\pm$ 0.3 v 4.8 $\pm$ 0.4; p $<$ 0.01). Since the severity of left ventricular damage is the major prognostic factor for late cardiac mortality, we would expect long-term survival for patients having thrombolysis to be improved in addition to the improvement in short-term survival.

The interrupted line in Fig. 2 shows that we have the reasonable expectation that hospital mortality rate for patients under 70 years of age who have thrombolysis can be reduced to 5% in 1987. When compared with the greater than 20% hospital mortality

rate which was reported almost universally before introduction of
Coronary Care Units in the 1960's, this rate must surely be
considered a remarkable achievement in public health terms. It is
very hard indeed to escape the conclusion that better treatment of
myocardial infarction and now coronary thrombosis must be playing a
continuing part in the decline in mortality from coronary heart
disease that has occurred in many countries over the last 20 years.

## CAN THE ACUTE MORTALITY BE REDUCED FURTHER?

I believe that it is necessary to place an increasing part of
our effort into applying what we know already, namely better public
education on the symptoms and natural history of heart attack, more
delegation of diagnosis and treatment to paramedics, and more
immediate transfer to the Coronary Care Unit of patients referred to
the hospital with chest pain and ECG changes. In New Zealand the
National Heart Foundation has a "Heart Attack Action!" campaign which
is promulgated through the media. The purpose of this campaign is to
describe the symptoms of heart atack, to advise the public to call an
ambulance and/or their general practitioner if they have cardiac pain
of more than 15 minutes duration, and to teach cardiopulmonary
resuscitation to the general public. In Auckland we have a well
organized life-support ambulance system with 6 units which are well
placed to serve a population of approximately 900,000 people and have
a delay in an emergency situation of about 8 minutes. Each
life-support unit carries a portable ECG machine, and we have taught
Advanced Care Ambulance Officers to diagnose ST segment changes from
the 12 lead ECG. Facilities are available to telemeter the ECG to
all four Coronary Care Units in Auckland and the Ambulance Officers
have been instructed to bring patients with chest pain and ST segment
changes directly to Coronary Care Units bypassing the Accident and
Emergency Departments.

I believe that in many hospitals, including our own, there is a
tendency to keep patients with myocardial infarctions longer in
Accident and Emergency than previously. A small study was conducted
by us (Gates R, Enwright JJ, Norris RM, manuscript in preparation) to
compare causes of such delays in 1985 with those in 1972. This study

showed that the delays attributable to patients reporting their symptoms in 1985 were identical with those in 1972. The "diagnostic delay" in making the decision on transfer of the patient to hospital had been reduced considerably, but hospital delay in the Accident and Emergency Department had increased by about one hour. This change had occurred because of the upgrading of Accident and Emergency Departments and the delegation of medical registrars to work solely in those Departments. Although there is an undoubted advantage in a pre-hospital work-up for the majority of patients who need diagnosis, it is clearly inappropriate for the patient who requires urgent thrombolysis.

In addition, we can almost certainly reduce hospital mortality further by use of more efficient methods for thrombolysis and possibly by the combined administration of a myocardial protective agent or agents together with the most effective thrombolytic drug. Information will soon be available on the comparative benefits of tissue plasminogen activator and streptokinase; administration of the thrombolytic agent by paramedics is a workable proposition which we hope to start in Auckland soon, and it is at least possible that an orally active thrombolytic agent will be developed which will decrease delay in initiation of thrombolysis even further. Furthermore, combined therapy with a thrombolytic and a myocardial protective agent is a logical extension of therapy and would be likely to reduce further myocardial ischaemic damage and hence mortality. We have shown that the combination of intravenous streptokinase with intravenous propranolol is well tolerated (11) and other myocardial supportive agents such as glucose-insulin-potassium and oxygen-free radical scavengers are well worthy of clinical trial and would be expected to be more effective in the presence of reperfusion than in the presence of permanent ischemia.

## LATE MORTALITY AFTER DISCHARGE FROM HOSPITAL

We have shown previously that 3 and 6 year mortality after infarction is related to the severity of the index infarction (as judged by the degree of cardiac enlargement and left ventricular failure assessed from the chest x-ray taken at the time of index

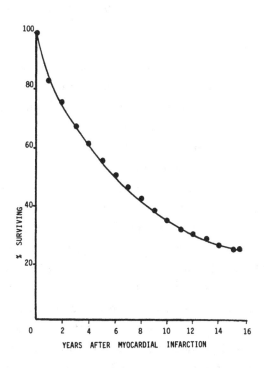

**FIGURE 5.** Survival of 530 patients (of all ages) after recovery from myocardial. Reprinted from Br. Med. J. (14) with permission.

infarct) and to the age of the patient (12,13). Surviving patients from this study which was conducted during 1966-67 were followed up again in 1982, giving a mean follow-up of 15 1/2 years with a 99% follow-up of patients alive at 6 years and a 95% follow-up overall (14). Increasing age, cardiac enlargement and congestion of the lung fields at the time of the index infarct continued to predict mortality between 6 and 15 years for patients who had survived to 6 years. Thus large infarct size, reflected by cardiac enlargement and impairment of left ventricular function, is likely to remain an increased risk factor even after recovery from infarction, for the rest of the patient's life. Fig. 5 shows the exponential curve after survival after index infarction in our study for patients of all ages and with all grades of severity, and Fig. 6 shows how cardiac enlargement remains a risk factor at 3, 6 and 15 years of follow-up.

## THE CORONARY ANATOMY

If long-term survival is indeed determined by the severity of the heart attack, could the severity of myocardial damage be most accurately quantified by invasive or non-invasive investigation after healing of the infarct? Could the severity of occlusions and stenoses of the coronary arteries, both of the infarct-related artery and of arteries supplying myocardium remote from the infarct, be additional risk factors? Between 1972 and 1984 we investigated two consecutive series of male patients under 60 years of age who had recovered from a first or recurrent myocardial infarct. Patients were studied after first infarction between 1977 and 1984 and after recurrent infarction between 1972 and 1979. A major aim of both of these studies was to conduct trials of coronary artery surgery in asymptomatic patients with advanced coronary disease. As the trials showed no difference in survival between surgically and conservatively treated patients (15) we were able to use the data for long-term prediction of prognosis on all 162 patients after recurrent infarction and 443 patients after first infarction in whom full angiocardiographic data had been obtained. This combined total of 605 patients represented more than 80% of consecutive cases passing through our Coronary Care Unit during these years, so there was minimum bias in selection of cases. Patients who had recurrent infarction had angiocardiography performed on average at two months after the infarct and patients with first infarction at one month after the event. Follow-up is continued annually at a special clinic, causes of death outside hospital are established from the patient's general practitioner or his relatives, survival is estimated actuarially, and analysis of risk factors is performed using the Cox proportional hazards model (16).

The striking fact which emerges from this study (which we believe to be the largest study with the longest follow-up so far

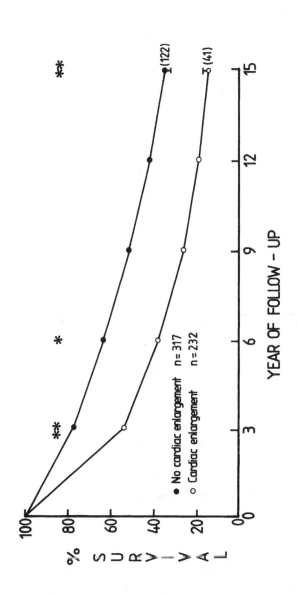

**FIGURE 6.** Effect of radiological cardiac enlargement at the time of the index infarct on 15 year survival. Patients of all ages are included. Vertical bars indicate SE's of estimates; figures at 15 years indicate numbers of survivors. Significance of differences among all age groups for survival up to 3 years, from 3 to 6 years and from 6 to 15 years; * p < 0.05; ** p < 0.01. Reprinted from the Br. Med. J. (14) with permission.

reported), is that on both univariate and on multivariate analysis survival appears to depend solely on the severity of left ventricular dysfunction and little if at all on the severity of coronary arterial disease. This is shown in Figs. 7 and 8. Although on univariate analysis there was a trend towards lower survival for patients with more severe coronary disease as evidenced by a high coronary score value (17) this difference disappeared on multivariate analysis. These results, although at first sight unexpected, should not be taken to mean that the untreated severity of coronary arterial lesions does not affect prognosis. Fifteen percent of the patients in the series shown in Figs. 6 and 7 had correction of their disordered coronary anatomy by coronary vein grafting which was done electively either for left main coronary stenosis or for relief of disabling post-infarction angina. A further 9% of the patients had

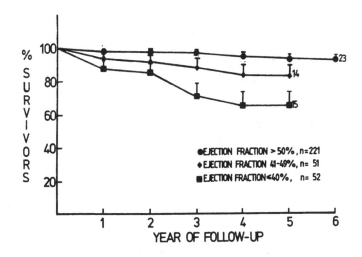

**FIGURE 7.** Actuarial survival curves according to the ejection fraction for 324 male patients under 60 years who had survived a first myocardial infarction. Numbers and bars are as described for Figure 6. The 3 curves are significantly different ($x_2$ = 34.0; p < 0.001). Reprinted from Amer. J. Cardiol. (18) with permission.

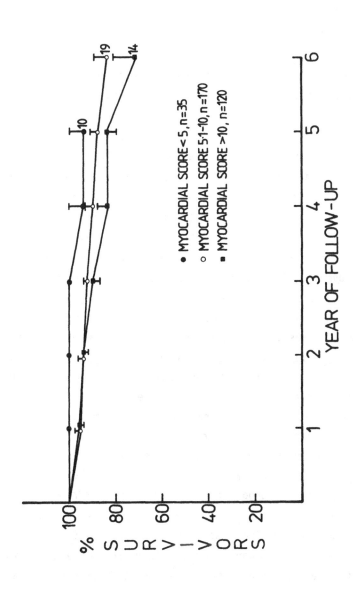

**FIGURE 8.** Actuarial survival curves according to the severity of coronary arterial occlusions and stenoses assessed by a scoring system (myocardial score; ref 17). Numbers and bars are as described for Figure 6. The curves are not significantly different $x_2 = 2.2$; $p < 0.3$). Reprinted from Amer. J. Cardiol. (18) with permission.

surgery as part of the randomized trial, but as the survival of these patients did not differ from those of the control patients who had similar coronary anatomy but did not have surgery, it is unlikely that surgery affected survival for this subset. Thus our data seem to show that the severity of coronary occlusions and stenoses is not an added risk factor provided the stenoses do not cause symptoms or involve the left main coronary artery, a conclusion which is supported by our own previous work (18) and by the results of the CASS Study (19).

If the severity of coronary arterial stenoses is not an independent risk factor for subsequent cardiac mortality is it a risk factor for subsequent reinfarction? We addressed this question in our patients after first infarction by following them for a mean period of 3.5 years during which time 40 patients had recurrent fatal or non-fatal infarcts (18). Although the "stenosis score" (proportion of left ventricular myocardium supplied by arteries having a hemodynamically significant stenosis) was significantly higher in the patients who had reinfarction during follow-up than those who did not, the range of stenosis score (from 0 - 100% in both groups of patients) was so wide that prediction of reinfarction for any individual patient from a high stenosis score would have been almost completely without value. Subsequently it has been shown that the anatomy of the stenosis rather than its severity is the factor which is associated with coronary thrombosis and infarction (20) and it remains to be seen whether presence of an eccentric irregular lesion as described by Ambrose and his colleagues can be used to predict infarction from coronary angiograms in the same way as it can be used to diagnose the probability of a coronary thrombosis in retrospect.

There is one interesting observation, however, which we have been able to make on coronary arterial anatomy in relation to prognosis, and it relates to patency of the infarct-related artery at four weeks after infarction. In a survey of 277 male patients from the first coronary project (21), my colleage Dr. Harvey White found that 75 (27%) of these patients, all of whom had had Q wave infarctions and none of whom had been treated with thrombolytic agents, anticoagulants, or antiplatelet drugs, had a patent infarct-related artery at the time of the four week angiogram. These patients had significantly higher ejection fractions and significantly longer survival over a mean follow-up of 44 months than those who had an occluded infarct-related artery. It was of particular interest that reinfarction was only slightly more common in patients who had a patent infarct-related artery than in those in whom it was occluded (11% vs 7%, not significant). Although a number of interpretations of this observation are possible, perhaps the most likely interpretation is that patients with patent infarct-related arteries had had spontaneous reperfusion, which resulted in improved left ventricular function and consequently in improved prognosis. If this interpretation is correct, it would be a further argument in favour of assisting the natural thrombolytic process at the the earliest possible time after the onset of coronary thrombosis.

## RESIDUAL LEFT VENTRICULAR FUNCTION

Although the ejection fraction is considered to be a reliable index of left ventricular function after infarction, there may be advantages in describing function in terms of left ventricular end-systolic volume. Fig. 9 shows two ventriculograms both taken in the right anterior oblique position of two patients, both of whom had ejection fractions of 29%. However, the two patients achieved the same ejection fraction to a markedly different end-systolic volume which was 230 ml in patient A and 117 ml in patient B. Patient A died suddenly after one month of follow-up while patient B survives after 8 years. Recently we have repeated the multivariate analysis of the clinical and arteriographic risk factor data on all patients studied after first or recurrent infarction, numbering 605 in all (22). The difference from our earlier analysis (18) is that we have considered end-systolic volume and end-diastolic volume in addition to ejection fraction in the multivariate analysis and we have widened the data base by adding data from the patients after recurrent infarction to those from the patients after first infarction which we had described previously. Log rank testing showed that end-systolic volume ($x_2$ = 82.9) had greater predictive value for survival than

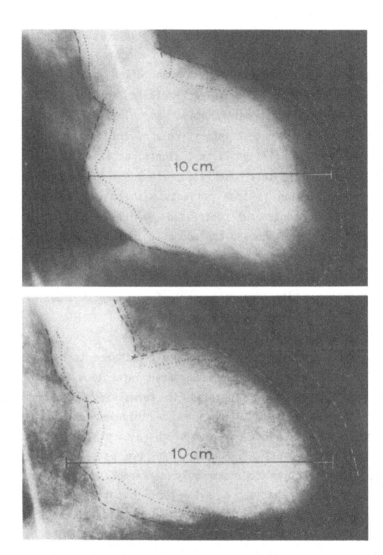

**FIGURE 9.** End-diastolic frames from left ventriculograms taken in the RAO projection of 2 patients with the same ejection fraction but markedly different end-systolic volumes (see text for details). Data suggest that prognosis is significantly worse for a given ejection fraction when end-systolic volume is very high (Patient A) than when it is only moderately increased (Patient B), and that end-systolic volume is a more accurate indicator of prognosis than ejection fraction. Note the thinned aneurysmal scar in Patient A and the normal myocardial wall thickness (distance between inner and outer lines) in Patient B. These lines indicate the endocardial and epicardial surfaces at end-systole (dotted lines) and end-diastole (broken lines).

end-diastolic volume ($x_2$ = 59), ejection fraction ($x_2$ = 46), or the severity of coronary occlusions ($x_2$ = 10). It should be noted that the severity of coronary stenoses as opposed to occlusions, second versus first infarction, age (for this restricted group of patients under 60 years of age), and whether or not the patient had had coronary surgery, had no predictive power, even on univariate analysis. When the factors were analyzed between survival and end-systolic volume and the square of end-systolic volume had been fitted, there was no additional significant predictive information in either end-diastolic volume or ejection fraction. Addition of the square of end-systolic volume to end-diastolic volume meant that the line expressing the relationship between these two variables was curvilinear with a disproportionate increase in the risk of cardiac death with increasing end-systolic volume.

## TRENDS FOR THE FUTURE

Is long-term prognosis after myocardial infarction improving? If so is it improving to the same degree as hospital mortality is declining? I should like to close this presentation with some preliminary data based on the survey by J.R. Fraser which I referred to earlier of chest x-rays from 400 patients with myocardial infarction admitted to Auckland hospitals during 1981. These patients were part of the Auckland ARCOS Study which was an epidemiological survey carried out by Dr. Robert Beaglehole and his colleagues from the Auckland University School of Medicine (23). Knowledge of the chest x-ray appearances on admission to hospital together with the patients' age and whether or not the infarct was the first or a recurrent infarct allowed us to calculate the coronary prognostic index for long-term survival (12) for these patients and to compare their 3 year survival with that of the original cohort of patients who had been discharged from hospital during 1966-67. We found that patients discharged during 1981 had had more severe infarcts, as assessed by the Coronary Prognostic Index, than those discharged during 1966-67. Despite this, 3 year survival had improved significantly (p < 0.01) from 75% for 1966-67 to 86% for 1981.

## SUMMARY AND CONCLUSIONS

Hospital mortality from acute myocardial infarction continues to fall and a mortality rate of 5% for patients under 70 years of age is now a reasonable expectation. The fall in mortality started with the introduction of Coronary Care Units, fell steadily during the 1970's and should fall further with more general use of thrombolytic therapy. It is difficult to escape the conclusion that some at least of the decline in mortality from coronary heart disease is due to improved management of acute myocardial infarction. After recovery from infarction the major prognostic factors are age and the functional status of the left ventricle, the latter being best described by end-systolic volume. The severity of coronary arterial stenoses after recovery from infarction does not appear to predict cardiac mortality and it is a poor guide to the risk of reinfarction provided patients with disabling post-infarction angina and those with left main coronary stenosis receive surgical treatment. Patency of the infarct-related artery after recovery from transmural infarction appears to be a favorable prognostic sign.

## REFERENCES

1. Norris, R.M., Brandt, P.W.T, Caughey, D.E., et al. Lancet i: 274-278, 1969.
2. Norris, R.M., Brandt, P.W.T, Lee, A.J. Lancet i: 278-281, 1969.
3. Norris, R.M., Sammel, N. Progr. Cardiovasc. Dis. 23: 129-140, 1980.
4. Norris, R.M., Brown, M.A., Clarke, E.D., et al. Lancet ii: 883-886, 1984.
5. ISIS-1 Collaborative Group. Lancet ii: 57-66, 1986.
6. GISSI Collaborative Group. Lancet i: 397-401, 1986.
7. ISAM Study Group. New Engl. J. Med. 314: 1465-1471, 1986.
8. Simmons, M.L., Brand, M. V/D, de Zwaan, C., et al. Lancet ii: 578-581, 1985.
9. Martin, G.V., Staduis, M.L., Davis, K.B., et al. Circulation 74 (Suppl. II): 367, 1986.
10. Kennedy, J.W., Ritchie, J.L., Davis, K.B., Fritz, J.K. New Engl. J. Med. 309: 1477-1482, 1983.
11. White, H., Brown, M., Takayama, M., et al. Circulation: 74 (Suppl II): 5, 1986.
12. Norris, R.M., Caughey, D.E., Mercer, C.J., et al. Lancet ii: 485-488, 1970.
13. Norris, R.M., Caughey, D.E., Mercer, P.J., Scott, P.J. Br. Heart J. 36: 786-790, 1974.

14. Merrilees, M.A., Scott, P.J., Norris, R.M. Br. Med. J. 288: 356-359, 1984.
15. Norris, R.M., Agnew, T.M., Brandt, P.W.T., et al. Circulation 63: 785-792, 1981.
16. Cox, D.R. J. Roy. Statist. Soc. B34: 187, 1972.
17. Brandt, P.W.T., Partridge, J.B., Wattie, W.J. Clin. Radiol. 28: 361-365, 1977.
18. Norris, R.M., Barnaby, P.F., Brandt, P.W.T., et al. Am. J. Cardiol. 53: 408-413, 1984.
19. CASS Principal Investigators et al. Circulation 68: 939-950, 1983.
20. Ambrose, J.A., Winter, L., Arora, R.R., et al. J. Am. Coll. Cardiol. 6: 1233, 1985.
21. White, H., Brown, M., Brandt, P., Norris, R. NZ Med. J. 98: 910, 1985.
22. White, H.D., Norris, R.M., Brown, M.A., et al. Circulation: In Press.
23. Beaglehole, R., Bonita, R., Jackson, R., et al. Am. J. Epidemiol. 120: 225-235, 1984.

# II. ASSESSMENT OF FUNCTION

# 5

## PHYSIOLOGICAL RESPONSE TO EXERCISE

Shepherd, R.F.J. and Shepherd J.T.

Mayo Clinic and Foundation, Rochester MN  55905

### INTRODUCTION

The performance of muscular exercise, either rhythmic (isotonic) or static (isometric), demands complex local, nervous and humoral adjustments of the cardiovascular system in order to meet the metabolic demands of the active muscles.  These adjustments of the heart, resistance and capacitance vessels and present knowledge of the mechanisms involved are summarized in this paper.

### LOCAL VASODILATION IN ACTIVE MUSCLES

The blood flow to the skeletal muscles, like that of other organs, depends primarily on the caliber of the resistance vessels and the perfusion pressure.  The muscles of the human body constitute about 45% of the body mass.  At rest, the total flow to them is about 1.2 liters/min, whereas during heavy exercise it may reach 20 liters/min in sedentary subjects and 40 liters/min in athletes (1). With maximal dynamic exercise of the knee extensors of one limb, the muscle flow is at least 200 ml/100 g/min (2).

During muscular contraction, chemical substances formed by the metabolically active skeletal muscles alter the tone of the resistance vessels in their vicinity.  These metabolites regulate locally the blood flow in proportion to the metabolic demands (Fig. 1).  This phenomenon is the link between oxygen needs and supply. While earlier studies sought to identify a single substance that could explain the exercise hyperemia, a single metabolic factor that is a universal mediator in all the muscles of all species is unlikely.  Present evidence seems to support a multifactorial metabolic control system that may vary from one species to another and even within a species depending on the severity and type of exercise. Thus $K^+$ release, hyperosmolarity, adenosine and adenine nucleotides in addition to other substances may all be involved (3,4).

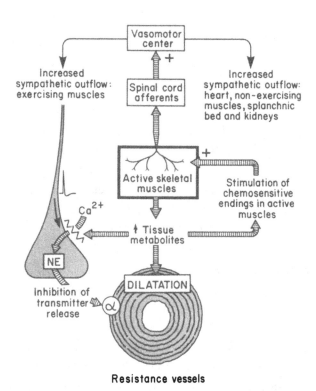

**Resistance vessels**

**FIGURE 1.** Cardiovascular changes due to contraction of skeletal muscles. Local metabolic products relax resistance vessels in active muscles and inhibit the output of norepinephrine from the sympathetic nerves in these muscles. Chemosensitive endings activated by metabolic products cause a reflex increase in sympathetic outflow to the heart, and systemic resistance and capacitance vessels. As a consequence an appropriate arterial blood pressure is achieved. As the strength of the muscle contraction increases, the blood flow to these muscles is mechanically impeded during the contractions. During isometric contractions, there is a greater activation of the chemosensitive endings and together with other factors, leads to a marked increase in arterial blood pressure.

The dilatation of the resistance blood vessels in the active muscles is accompanied by an increase in the diameter of the large inflow arteries. Studies on isolated arteries suggest that this change in the large inflow arteries is due to a flow dependent release of a relaxing factor from the endothelial cells (5,6).

During rhythmic exercise, as the force of contraction increases with increasing severity of exercise, the blood flow is mechanically impeded during the contraction. Thus, similar to that of the heart muscle, the maximal flow is achieved in the intervals between the contractions. During strong isometric exercise, the impedance is continuous. The greater increase in arterial blood pressure during isometric exercise helps to some extent to maintain the perfusion of the contracted muscles (see later).

## INCREASE IN CARDIAC OUTPUT

In humans resting supine in a comfortable environment, the stress on the cardiovascular system is minimal because the metabolic requirements of the body and gravitational and thermal stresses are small. The heart rate is mainly under vagal restraint. During leg exercise in this position, the cardiac output increases due to an increase in heart rate with no change or a 10-20% increase in the stroke volume due to greater left ventricular emptying (7). The increase in heartrate occurs through a simultaneous decrease in vagal activity and an increase in the output of norepinephrine from the sympathetic nerve endings acting on $beta_1$-adrenoceptors on the sinus node, and on the atrioventricular node and conducting tissue to shorten the refractory period and enhance myocardial contractility (Fig. 2). With increasing age the response to $beta_1$-adrenergic stimulation in man is attenuated. However, despite the smaller increase in heart rate and ventricular contractility, an increase in end-diastolic volume and stroke volume compensates (8). Coronary blood flow during exercise is increased in proportion to the work of the heart, due to the action of local metabolic products such as adenosine on coronary resistance vessels. The norepinephrine released at the sympathetic nerve endings on the coronary vessels acts predominantly on $beta_1$-adrenoceptors to cause vasodilatation.

This effect enhances the metabolically induced relaxation (9).

When a supine subject stands <u>upright</u> in a relaxed manner, 300-800 ml additional blood is contained in the legs and the cardiac volume decreases by about 20%. The hydrostatic shift of blood results in a marked decrease in cardiopulmonary blood volume, filling pressure of the heart and stroke volume. As a result the cardiac output is reduced by about 1.0 - 1.7 liters/min (10). To maintain an adequate arterial blood pressure under these circumstances requires an increase in systemic vascular resistance and an overall diminution in capacity of the systemic venous system (Fig. 2) (11).

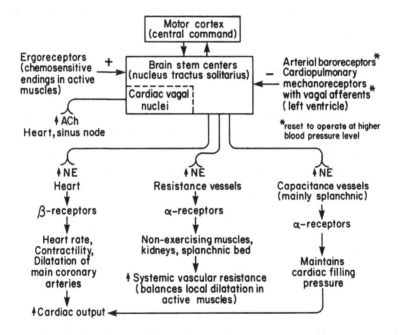

**FIGURE 2.** Key mechanisms involved in the autonomic nervous adjustments of the cardiovascular system during muscular exercise. ACh = acetylcholine;  NE = norepinephrine.

The main reflexes involved in maintaining circulatory homeostasis in the upright position are mediated by the arterial baroreceptors and the mechanoreceptors in the heart and lungs subserved by vagal afferents (12). Ergoreceptors in the skeletal muscles of the legs, activated by the tensing of these muscles on standing, may contribute to these reflex adjustments.

In the early moments of standing, there is an immediate increase in heart rate caused by withdrawal of cardiac vagal activity. There follows a further rate increase and an abrupt decrease accompanied by opposite changes in arterial blood pressure. An initial decrease in arterial blood pressure is caused by the rapid reduction in cardiac output. This reduction is due to the rapid translocation of blood from the thorax prior to the increase in sympathetic outflow to the systemic resistance and capacitance vessels (13,14). On transition from rest to exercise, the action of the leg muscle pump redistributes the blood centrally so that the intrathoracic blood volume and stroke volume approach their supine values (7). With increasing dynamic upright exercise, the stroke volume and heart rate have a similar pattern to that during supine exercise. The cardiac output increases by 5 - 6 litres/min for each 1 liter/min increase in oxygen uptake (15).

In normal humans, the upper limit of rhythmic exercise is determined by the cardiovascular system, since ventilation, gas diffusion in the lungs and gas exchange in the capillary beds of the active muscles do not limit performance. However, whereas sedentary normal subjects utilize about two thirds of their pulmonary capacity, in champion athletes the cardiovascular and pulmonary oxygen transport capacity are closely matched, indicating that in these circumstances pulmonary function may contribute as a limiting factor (1).

## EFFECT OF SYMPATHETIC BLOCKADE

After induction of beta-adrenergic blockade the heart rate during exercise is less than in normal subjects and the increase in cardiac contractility is attenuated. However, while the capacity for strenuous exercise is reduced, other mechanisms can compensate during milder exercise (16,17). In healthy subjects beta-blocking drugs do not alter the neural release of norepinephrine during exercise and have little effect on the release of epinephrine (18). By using M-mode echocardiography, it has been shown that beta-blockade in healthy subjects during semisupine exercise increased the end-diastolic dimension and systolic myocardial shortening (19).

Studies in dogs exercising after complete surgical denervation of the heart have shown that there is little limitation in their maximal capacity for exercise. They compensate for the lesser heart rate increase by a greater stroke volume and also by the "supersensitivity" of the cardiac $beta_1$-adrenoceptor to circulating norepinephrine (20,21). The same mechanism appears to operate in man (22). Some of the increase in heart rate after cardiac denervation is attributable to basic mechanisms intrinsic to the heart (23).

## ROLE OF RESISTANCE VESSELS IN SYSTEMIC VASCULAR BEDS OUTSIDE THE ACTIVE MUSCLES

To maintain arterial blood pressure and hence the perfusion pressure to help compensate for the decrease in systemic vascular resistance as the local metabolites dilate the resistance vessels in the active skeletal muscles, there is an increase in sympathetic outflow proportional to the work load. This causes constriction of the resistance vessels in the splanchnic bed and kidneys. The degree of dilatation caused by the local metabolites and the constrictor drive from the sympathetic outflow acting on alpha-adrenoreceptors on the systemic vessels is proportional to the intensity of the exercise and to the magnitude of the active muscle mass (15). In the working muscles the sympathetic control is nullified probably as a consequence of local metabolic products reducing the output of norepinephrine from the sympathetic nerve endings (Fig. 1) (24). Thus, an increase in hydrogen or potassium ions, or in osmolarity, can inhibit the exocytotic release of norepinephrine, possibly by depressing the entry of calcium ions into the nerve endings. This local modulation of norepinephrine release ensures that working muscles are perfused according to their needs while non-working muscles and the kidney and splanchnic bed provide a compensatory increase in vascular resistance. Thus the increase in cardiac output is available for the active muscles while an appropriate perfusion pressure is maintained.

In the early stages of heart failure, a decreased stroke volume is compensated for by relative tachycardia so that cardiac output is normal at submaximal levels of exercise. In patients with severe heart failure the heart rate and cardiac output response is compromised. There is, at the same work load as normal subjects, a greater constriction of the resistance vessels in vascular beds outside the active muscles, due to a greater reflex activation of the sympathetic nerves. This serves to redistribute the limited cardiac output to the vital organs and to maintain arterial blood pressure (25). However, the resultant increase in afterload imposes a further burden on the heart. It may be that, due to the reduced cardiac output, the chemoreceptors in the active muscles are activated earlier in these patients.

When patients with chronic idiopathic autonomic failure engage in mild supine leg exercise, their arterial blood pressure decreases even though the cardiac output increases normally. This decrease is due to a failure of reflex constriction of systemic vessels to compensate for the vasodilation in the active leg muscles (26). Even the ingestion of food in these patients may cause a fall in arterial pressure probably due to splanchnic vasodilatation, not compensated by an increase in sympathetic outflow (27).

## ROLE OF CAPACITANCE VESSELS

The increased sympathetic outflow during exercise causes constriction of the splanchnic capacitance vessels with active mobilization of blood from the veins of the liver, spleen and intestines. This change, together with passive mobilization resulting from constriction of the resistance vessels in the kidney and splanchnic bed provide an adequate filling pressure of the heart and hence maintenance or an increase in stroke volume. In the upright position the muscle pump in the legs is an important contributor to the filling pressure. During prolonged exercise the hemoglobin concentration of the blood increases consequent to a decrease in plasma volume resulting from the augmented exudation of fluid in the dilated muscle bed. The oxygen carry capacity of the blood is increased thereby.

## EXERCISE IN A HOT ENVIRONMENT

The thermoregulatory effector mechanisms are controlled by receptors in the skin, sensitive to cold and to heat and by central thermoreceptors in the hypothalamus, brain stem and spinal cord.

The heat generated by the active muscles causes the temperature of the blood to increase with resulting dilatation of the skin vessels and sweating. The increase in skin blood flow necessitates a further increase in cardiac output and greater constriction of the resistance vessels in the kidney and the splanchnic bed and of the splanchnic capacitance vessels. During severe heat stress the total skin flow may increase from about 0.2 liters/min to about 7 liters/min (28).

## HORMONAL AGENTS

Both plasma norepinephrine and epinephrine are increased in proportion to the intensity and duration of dynamic exercise (29). There are $beta_2$-adrenoceptors in the skeletal muscle resistance vessels which are not innervated by sympathetic nerves. Their function is unknown. While they can be activated by circulating epinephrine, they are not necessary for the increase in flow to the active muscles. Thus local beta-blockade of these vessels does not interfere with the increase in blood flow to these muscles during exercise (30, 31).

During dynamic exercise the plasma norepinephrine level is higher in subjects with borderline hypertension than in normotensives. It is suggested that this may be a consequence of less efficient baroreflexes in patients with hypertension (32, 33).

Plasma renin activity is decreased at rest and exercise by beta-blockers. However, there is no evidence that circulating angiotension II is necessary for the normal response to exericse (34).

## ROLE OF CARDIOVASCULAR REFLEXES

### Arterial baroreflexes

During both rhythmic and isometric exercise in man the carotid baroreceptors are adjusted rapidly to a higher level (Fig. 2). This "resetting" assists the arterial blood pressure to increase to help meet the metabolic demands of the active muscles. The shapes of the curves relating the changes in carotid sinus pressure to the systemic arterial pressure and to the heart rate are unchanged. Thus exercise does not diminish the overall gain of the carotid sinus baroreflex (35). Studies in dogs have shown that the arterial baroreflexes control the total systemic vascular resistance during and after exercise. When their influence is acutely withdrawn, the arterial pressure decreases more at the onset of exercise, rises excessively after exercise and remains elevated for a longer time after exercise ceases. By contrast heart rate and cardiac output increase normally during exercise, indicating that other mechanisms are responsible for the heart rate and cardiac output changes (36, 37). These may be the ergoreceptors in the skeletal muscles and the participation of the higher brain centers during exercise.

Cardiopulmonary mechanoreceptors

On standing upright in a relaxed manner, the shift of blood to the lower parts of the body decreases the signal both to the arterial and to the cardiopulmonary mechanoreceptors subserved by vagal afferents, with a resultant increase in sympathetic outflow to the heart, systemic resistance and capacitance vessels, adrenal medulla and juxtaglomerular cells of the kidney. There follows an increase in heart rate, a decrease in stroke volume, a reflex constriction of muscle, splanchnic and renal resistance vessels and splanchnic capacitance vessels and an increase in plasma renin activity. When the generation of angiotension II from renin is prevented by the administration of converting enzyme inhibitor, sodium-replete subjects can maintain their arterial blood pressure during an upright tilt, whereas in sodium-depleted subjects there is a decrease in systolic and diastolic pressure (38). In dogs, the cardiopulmonary receptors cannot prevent the excessive rise in arterial blood pressure with exercise after acute abrogation of the arterial baroreflex. However, after chronic denervation of the arterial baroreceptors, they are necessary to restore the total systemic vascular resistance to the resting value at the end of exercise (39).

In highly trained young athletes, the gain of the

cardiopulmonary receptor reflex in control of forearm vascular resistance is greater than in age-matched nonathletes (40).

Sympathetic Veno-Arteriolar Reflex

The increase in venous pressure in the lower limbs during head-up tilt or standing relaxed activates a local sympathetic veno-arteriolar reflex. This reflex, together with a direct myogenic response of the resistance vessels to the increased transmural pressure contributes to the peripheral vasoconstriction on assuming the upright posture and hence to the maintenance of arterial blood pressure (41). It is estimated that about half of the tilt-induced increase in vasoconstriction in the lower part of the body may be ascribed to the local venoarteriolar reflex (42).

Ergoreceptors

A strong static contraction of the skeletal muscles or a rapid powerful rhythmic contraction causes a marked increase in arterial blood pressure. The receptors in the muscles which cause the increase in sympathetic outflow and hence the hemodynamic changes appear to be activated by the product of muscle metabolism whereas those that cause the accompanying increase in heart rate might be governed by muscle receptors sensitive to changes in tension. The sensory fibers involved are the small myelinated (Group III) and unmyelinated (Group IV) afferents (43).

In addition to the reflex from the active muscles, there is a "central command" from the cerebral cortex to the cardiovascular centers in the brain stem (Fig. 2). It is suggested that this central command has the key role in causing the tachycardia, and the muscle chemosensitive endings in causing the increase in sympathetic outflow to the systemic vessels. Thus both mechanisms aid the increase in arterial blood pressure, and are not truly redundant (43,44).

The increase in arterial blood pressure is caused by the augmented sympathetic outflow and is due both to an increase in cardiac output and in systemic vascular resistance. If the output does not increase normally, there is increased constriction of the systemic resistance vessels so that the same rise in arterial pressure occurs. The prime purpose of the reflex seems to be to increase the blood flow to the contracting muscles. By an unknown means, presumably central, the arterial and the cardiopulmonary mechanoreceptors are rendered unable to oppose the increase in blood pressure (44, 35).

While it may appear that the characteristic hemodynamic change during static exercise is the arterial pressor response and that during dynamic exercise it is a volume response, similar mechanisms are involved in the complex circulatory adjustments to both types, including the ergoreceptors, central command, alterations in the set-point of the arterial and cardiopulmonary mechanoreflexes, circulating substances and local metabolic factors. Thus heart rate and systolic blood pressure are similar during static and dynamic exercise of identical muscle groups at equivalent work loads and persist after beta-adrenergic and parasympathetic blockade. Stroke volume and cardiac output are higher during dynamic than during static exercise of identical muscle groups carried to fatigue. Also plasma norpinephrine is higher during dynamic exercise, and total systemic vascular resistance is lower. These differences, however, reflect quantitative rather than qualitative differences in the response, due to different metabolic conditions in the active muscles and the prolonged mechanical compression of the vessels with severe isometric exercise (15).

## REFERENCES
1. Blomqvist, C.G., Saltin, B. Ann. Rev. Physiol. 45: 169-189, 1983.
2. Anderson, P., Saltin, B. J. Physiol. 366: 233-249, 1985.
3. Sparks, H.V. Fed. Proc. 39: 1487-1490, 1980.
4. Shepherd, J.T. Handbook of Physiology. Sect. 2. The Cardiovascular System, Vol. III. Peripheral Circulation and Organ Blood Flow. Part I, 319-370, 1983. Amer. Physiol. Soc. Williams and Wilkins, Baltimore.
5. Smiesko, V., Kozik, J., Dolezel, S. Blood Vessels 22: 247-251, 1985.
6. Rubanyi, G.M., Romero, J.C., Vanhoutte, P.M. Amer. J. Phsyiol. 250 (Heart Circ. Physiol. 19) H1145-H1149, 1986.
7. Bevegord, B.S., Shepherd, J.T. Physiol. Rev. 47: 178-212, 1967.
8. Rodeheffer, R.J., Gerstenblith, G., Becker, L.C., et al. Circulation 69: 203-213, 1984.
9. Cohen, R.A., Shepherd, J.T., Vanhoutte, P.M. Circ. Res. 52: 16-25, 1983.

10. Bevegord, B.S., Holmgren, A. , Jonsson, B. Acta. Physiol. Scand. 57: 26-50, 1963.
11. Shepherd, J.T. Alfred Benzon Symposium 23. Eds. Christensen, N.J., Henriksen, O., Lassen, N.A. Munksgaard, Copenhagen, p. 103-115, 1986.
12. Shepherd, J.T. Cardiovasc. Res. 16: 357-370, 1982.
13. Borst, C., Wieling, W., van Brederode, J.F.M., et al. Amer. J. Physiol. 243 (Heart Circ. Physiol. 12) H676-H681, 1982.
14. Borst, C., van Brederode, J.F.M., Wieling, W., et al. Clin. Sci. 67: 321-327, 1984.
15. Blomqvist, C.G., Lewis, S.F. Alfred Benzon Symposium 23. Eds. Christensen, N.J., Henriksen, O., Lassen, N.A. Munksgaard, Copenhagan, p. 188-199, 1986.
16. Epstein, S.E., Robinson, B.F., Kahler, R.L., Braunwald, E.J. Clin. Invest. 44: 1745, 1753, 1965.
17. Donald, D.E., Ferguson, D.A., Milburn, S.E. Circ. Res. 22: 127-134, 1968.
18. Sheehan, M.W., Brammell, H.L., Sable, D.L., et al. Amer. Heart J. 105: 777-782, 1983.
19. Anderson, K., Vik-Mo, H. Br. Heart J. 48: 149-155, 1982.
20. Donald D.E., Shepherd J.T. Amer. J. Cardiol. 14: 853-859, 1964.
21. Shepherd, J.T. Amer. J. Cardiol. 55: 87D-94D, 1985.
22. Bexton, R.S., Milne, J.R., Cory-Pearce, R., et al. Br. Heart J. 49: 584-588, 1983.
23. Donald, D.E., Samueloff, S.L. Am. J. Physiol. 211: 703-711, 1966.
24. Shepherd, J.T., Vanhoutte, P.M. J. Cardiovasc. Pharmacol. 7: S167-S178, 1985.
25. Francis, G.S., Goldsmith, S.R., Ziesche, S.M., Cohn, J.N. Amer. J. Cardiol. 49: 1152-1156, 1982.
26. Marshall, R.J., Schirger, A., Shepherd, J.T. Circulation 24: 76-81, 1961.
27. Mathias, C.J., da Costa, D.F., Fosbraey, P., et al. Alfred Benzon Symposium 23. Eds. Christensen, N.J., Henriksen, O., Lassen, N.A. Munksgaard, Copenhagen, p. 401-419, 1986.
28. Rowell, L.B. Handbook of Physiology, Sect. I. The Cardiovascular System, Vol. III, pt. 2, Amer. Physiol. Soc. Williams and Wilkins, Washington, D.C. p. 967-1024, 1983.
29. Christensen, N.J., Galbo, H. Ann. Rev. Physiol. 45: 139-153, 1983.
30. Hartling, O.J., Noer, I., Svendsen, T.L., et al. Clin. Sci. 58: 279-286, 1980.
31. Juhlin-Dannfelt, A., Aström, H. Scand. J. Clin. Lab. Invest. 39: 179-183, 1979.
32. Klein, A.A., McCrory, W.W., Engle, M.A., et al. J. Amer. Coll. Cardiol. 3: 381-386, 1984.
33. Sleight, P., Floras J.S., Hassan, M.O., et al. Clin. Sci. 57: 169s-171s, 1979.
34. McLeod, A.A., Brown, J.E., Kuhn, C., et al. Circulation 67: 1076-1084, 1983.
35. Shepherd, J.T., Mancia, G. Rev. Physiol. Biochem. Pharmacol. 105: 1-99, 1986.
36. Walgenbach, S.C., Donald, D.E. Circ. Res. 52: 253-262, 1983.

37. Walgenbach, S.C., Shepherd, J.T.   Mayo Clinic Proceedings   59: 467-475, 1984.
38. Sancho, J., Re, R., Burton, J., et al.   Circulation   53: 400-405, 1976.
39. Daskalopoulos, D.A., Shepherd, J.T., Walgenbach, S.C.   J. Appl. Physiol: Respirat. Environ. Exercise Physiol. 57(5): 1417-1421, 1984.
40. Takeshita, A., Jingu, S., Imaizumi, T., et al.   Circ. Res.   59: 43-48, 1986.
41. Henriksen, O.   Alfred Benzon Symposium 23.   Eds. Christensen, N.J., Lassen, N.A.   Munksgaard, Copenhagen, p. 67-80, 1986.
42. Skagen, K., Henriksen, O.   Alfred Benzon Symposium 23.   Eds. Christensen, N.J., Lassen, N.A.   Munksgaard, Copenhagen, p. 95-101, 1986.
43. Mitchell, J.H., Schmidt, R.F.   Handbook of Physiology, Sect. 2, The Cardiovascular System, Vol. III, part 2. Am. Physiol. Soc. Williams and Wilkins, Washington, D.C.  p. 623-658, 1983.
44. Shepherd, J.T., Blomqvist, C.G., Lind, A.R., et al.   Circ. Res. Part II, Vol 48 (6) I-179 - I-188, 1981.
45. Mark, A.L., Victor, R.G., Nerhed, C., et al.   Adrenergic Physiology and Pathophysiology.   Eds. Christensen, N.S., Henriksen, O., Lassen N.A.   Alfred Benzon Foundation, Munksgaard, Copenhagen, p. 221-233, 1986.

# 6

## ASSESSMENT OF VENTRICULAR FUNCTION IN MAN

M.I.M. Noble*, A.J. Drake-Holland**, S. Parker*, C.J. Mills***, J.A. Innes****, S. Pugh****, N. Mehta**

*King Edward VII Hospital, Midhurst, W. Sussex GU29OBL, U.K., **Department of Medicine 1, St. George's Hospital Medical School, London, ***Cardiothoracic Institute, Midhurst, ****Department of Medicine, Charing Cross and Westminster Medical School

### INTRODUCTION

For the clinician following patients who have suffered myocardial infarction an assessment of ventricular function is an important part of clinical management. What is debatable is how extensively one needs to document the extent of ventricular function in order to manage patients adequately. For example, the widely used New York Heart Association Classification of Heart Failure allows us to at least put patients into Class I or IV very easily, although a lot of debate occurs over who goes into Class II or III. Similarly the use of diuretic drugs and other inotropic agents provide a satisfactory clinical assessment of progress and prognosis. In addition, commonly used indices of cardiac size such as from the bi-plane chest radiograph or echocardiographic dimensions also allow both clinically and prognostically useful information to be obtained. The question that we should ask is, "Would we obtain any more useful information by a more detailed assessment of ventricular function?" This question is important in the light of new more aggressive approaches to the management of patients after myocardial infarction where options might include coronary artery bypass grafting and possibly cardiac transplantation. In these cases it is important to have as accurate an assessment as possible of ventricular function in order to answer such fundamental questions as:

1. Is the patient's reserve of ventricular function so small as to merit consideration of immediate coronary artery bypass surgery even though his symptoms would not otherwise fulfill the usual criteria for surgery?

2. In the patient who has severe angina, previous coronary artery bypass surgery, and extensive previous myocardial infarction, is ventricular function sufficiently well preserved to allow the patient to withstand a further revascularization procedure, or should one wait for cardiac transplantation?

Besides what one might term static assessment, it is usual to perform some form of dynamic assessment such as exercise testing in order to further evaluate the patient's objective symptoms and myocardial performance.

Some patients after myocardial infarction will have angina and others may have evidence of ST segment depression consistent with ischemia during exercise. When evidence of ischemia is found, evidence of left ventricular function can usually be found also. Part of the assessment prior to coronary artery bypass surgery should involve assessment of ventricular function when the patient is not suffering myocardial ischemia, in order that the possible benefits of revascularization to areas of potentially ischemic myocardium can be evaluated. However, the level of exercise which is achieved before the ischemia develops varies significantly from patient to patient and there is no standard level of exercise at which measurements can be made. Under these circumstances, a resting measurement may be the most reliable index one can use for comparative purposes.

Because of the major difficulties of using exercise to assess ventricular function in the absence of ischemia in patients who have suffered prior myocardial infarction, we have concentrated upon indices which can be derived at rest. It is recognized that there would be many advantages in looking at exercise indices but the difficulties, some of which have been outlined above, have precluded a reliable index being developed up to the present time.

## INDICES OF CONTRACTILITY

On the basis of previous animal experimentation we have devised some ideas about a perfect index of contractility. These are

a. that it is insensitive to changes in arterial pressure and end diastolic volume,

b. it is responsive to changes in contractility,

c. in order to avoid confusion from reflex effects on heart rate and
blood pressure an attempt should be made to control these variables.

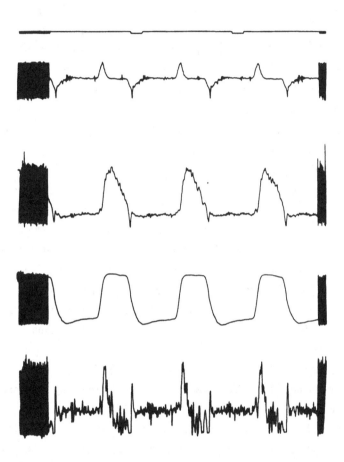

**FIGURE 1.** The second trace from the top is the primary record
obtained with the Mills electromagnetic velocity probe in the
ascending aorta, while the tip of the catheter records left
ventricular pressure with a tip manometer (Gaeltec, 3rd trace). Left
ventricular pressure and aortic velocity are differentiated
electronically to give LVdp/dt (top) and acceleration (bottom).

Our group has overcome some of these disadvantages by studying
the patients under adequate beta-adrenergic blockade and using right
atrial pacing to avoid any changes in heart rate, contractility and
blood pressure produced by sympathetic stimulation induced reflexly.

The only indices which are insensitive to changes in arterial pressure are those obtained in the isovolumic contraction period such as the maximum rate of rise of left ventricular pressure (LVdp/dtmax). This proposition is true as long as aortic pressure does not fall so low that this maximum cannot be reached before the aortic valve opens. All ejection indices are affected by arterial pressure; however, when the arterial pressure is constant, ejection indices can be considered.

In the cardiac catheterization laboratory we have measured the responses to an increase in end diastolic volume achieved by tilting. Left ventricular pressure was measured by a Gaeltec catheter tip manometer mounted on the same catheter as a Mills electromagnetic velocity transducer positioned in the ascending aorta (1). The heart rate was maintained constant by pacing the right atrium. Aortic cross-diameter was measured by 2D echocardiography. Stroke volume and cardiac output were calculated from the integral of aortic velocity and aortic cross-sectional area. Maximum acceleration of blood from the left ventricle was obtained by differentiation of velocity. LVdp/dtmax was obtained by differentiation of left ventricular pressure.

An example of the records obtained is given in Fig. 1. On a separate occasion, ejection fraction was obtained by radionuclide angiography. This value was assumed to apply to the resting control state during Mills probe catheterization. Control end diastolic volume was then calculated from ejection fraction and stroke volume. End systolic volume was assumed to be constant when end diastolic volume was increased (2) enabling us to calculate the change in ejection fraction from the measured stroke volume values.

It can be seen from the results shown in Fig. 2 that tilting from the head up to the head down position during cardiac catheterization provides an adequate change in end diastolic pressure and volume to test the effect on various indices of contractility (Fig. 3A). There is a variable but definite effect on all the ejection indices, namely stroke volume, cardiac output, ejection fraction, peak aortic blood velocity, and maximum acceleration of blood from the left ventricle. This last index is much more sensitive to end diastolic volume changes in man than in dog (3). LVdp/dtmax was almost completely unaffected by tilt under these circumstances of beta-adrenergic blockade and right atrial pacing. The small changes that did occur were variable in polarity. This behavior can be expected from theoretical considerations (3).

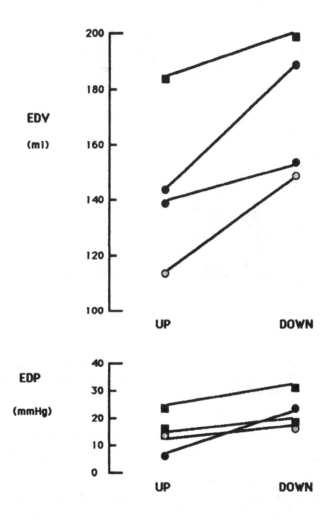

**FIGURE 2.** The effect of tilting 4 beta-blocked patients from head up to head down on LV end-diastolic volume (EDV) and end-diastolic pressure (EDP).

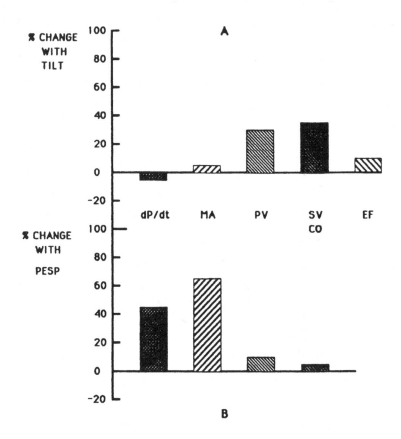

**FIGURE 3.** A. The effect of tilt as in Fig. 2 on variables of contraction. B. The effect of post-extrasystolic potentiation. Means from 4 patients shown in Fig. 2.

In order to test the sensitivity of these indices to a change in contractility, post extrasystolic potentiation was studied by appropriate irregular pacing patterns (Fig. 3B). From these results it is clear that LVdp/dtmax was the only completely satisfactory index of contractility. Therefore we recommend that when the question is asked "Does a particular therapeutic intervention affect contractility?", the answer should be obtained by measuring LVdp/dtmax under beta-adrenergic blockade and right atrial pacing at constant heart rate.

## WHAT IS THE BEST INDEX OF CONTRACTILITY IN ASSESSING OVERALL VENTRICULAR FUNCTION AFTER MYOCARDIAL INFARCTION?

Problems arise with most of the indices which have been used when trying to assess ventricular function after myocardial infarction. The reasons for this are that LVdp/dtmax is an isovolumic index which cannot reflect the pumping action of the heart, all of which takes place later in systole. Secondly, LVdp/dtmax depends not only upon contractility but also upon the synchonicity of contraction. This problem can be demonstrated very simply by recording the drop in LVdp/dtmax that occurs on switching from atrial pacing to ventricular pacing. Thus, LVdp/dtmax is reduced by bundle branch block and will also be affected by regional mechanical dysfunction secondary to previous infarction.

Therefore, although LVdp/dtmax is the best index to be measured in a given patient with constant synchroncity in assessing contractility changes, it is not an ideal index in the presence of ventricular dysfunction secondary to myocardial infarction.

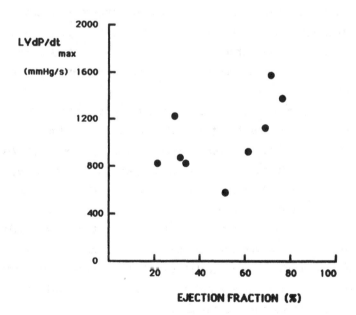

**FIGURE 4.** LVdp/dtmax measured at cardiac catheterization under beta-adrenergic blockade compared to ejection fraction by MUGA, measured on a separate occasion not under beta blockade.

Nevertheless, we have found in a small patient group a statistically significant correlation (Spearman Rank correlation coefficient, $r_s$ = 0.72) between LVdp/dtmax and an excellent and well accepted index of overall mechanical function, the ejection fraction (Fig. 4).

## THEORETICAL BASIS FOR EJECTION FRACTION AS AN ACCURATE INDEX OF OVERALL LEFT VENTRICULAR MECHANICAL FUNCTION

The sarcomere is the basic contractile unit of heart muscle. Its contractile function can be shown by a relationship between length and contractile force (4). The corresponding relationship for the intact left ventricle is that between volume and isovolumically developed pressure (2). The same relationship applies to the volume and pressure at the end of systole, provided that the duration of systole is long enough and the velocity of contraction is high enough for these values to be obtained before relaxation intervenes. These last two conditions shift the end systolic pressure volume curve to the right of the isovolumic curve indicating an apparent decrease in ventricular function. Since such curtailment of the duration of systole or the low velocity of contraction are abnormal, pathological and an indication of disease, the clinical usefulness of the end systolic pressure volume curve is no way lessened. Unfortunately, it is impossible to determine the isovolumic curve in man. It is also not practical to determine the end systolic pressure volume curve because accurate simultaneous measurements of left ventricular volume and pressure are required for this calculation, while the patient's systolic pressure is varied over a wide range. However, providing the patients are always studied with normal blood pressure, the position of the end systolic pressure volume curve is indicated by the ejection fraction as illustrated in Fig. 5. When the end systolic pressure volume curve shifts to the right as the result of decreased overall left ventricular mechanical function, there is a compensatory increase in end diastolic volume so that stroke volume is maintained (Fig. 5). However, the ratio of stroke volume to end diastolic volume (ejection fraction) declines.

We therefore conclude that the use of ejection fraction as the standard clinical index of ventricular function is well justified on theoretical grounds and should be the measurement with which alternative indices should be compared. There remains the question of the method of measurement. Left ventricular angiography is invasive and outlining of the cavity from films is a subjective process and liable to observer error, and the calculation of the ejection fraction also requires unwarranted assumptions about left ventricular geometry which may be particularly untrue in the case of the damaged ventricle secondary to previous infarction. More useful is the non-invasive nuclear method (MUGA). No assumption of ventricular geometry is made because the radioactive counts from the blood pool in the cavity are proportional to the volume of blood. The investigator is required to delineate the left ventricular cavity blood pool on the gamma camera image and to exclude right ventricular and atrial counts by patient positioning. Once this has been done, the measurement of ejection fraction is objective. However, there is some dispute about the problems of subtraction of background count and this has not been completely resolved.

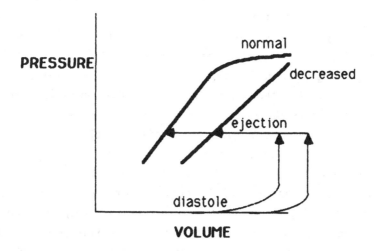

**FIGURE 5.** Schema of the effect of impairment of LV contraction on the end-systolic pressure/volume curve and ejection fraction.

## ARE THERE ANY OTHER INDICES WORTHY OF CONSIDERATION?

Ejection fraction is so commonly used (and is obtained fairly readily by non-invasive means), that one might ask the question should we look for anything else? However, nuclear medicine departments cannot be provided in many hospitals and this places restrictions on the number of patients and the frequency of measurements. Ideally, we would require a very simple, quick and non-invasive method that could be used in the physician's office as often as he wished and would allow repeated measurements over time. The possibility of this is being provided by the availability of transcutaneous doppler measurements of ascending aortic blood velocity (5) made from the suprasternal notch (6,7,8).

## AORTIC VELOCITY AND ACCELERATION VS. EJECTION FRACTION

On the basis of animal experiments in dogs in which large percentage falls in maximum acceleration were found following coronary artery occlusion (9) one might expect a concordance between the aortic acceleration and the ejection fraction. Bennett et al (10) attempted to validate this prediction by invasive measurements in man. This was performed using an ejection fraction obtained angiographically. A good correlation was found between the angiographically estimated ejection fraction and both peak velocity and maximum acceleration. Since that time the Mills probe has been improved by being made more sensitive and by being mounted on the shaft of the catheter, the tip of which is in the ventricle. This latter modification stablizes the position of the probe within the ascending aorta and reduces movement artefact, yielding traces of high quality (Fig. 1). With this method we were still able to obtain a good correlation between maximal acceleration and ejection fraction ($r_s$ = 0.73) but a less good correlation between peak velocity and ejection fraction ($r_s$ = 0.45). These correlations may have been reduced by the fact that the ejection fraction measurements were made on a different day in the absence of beta-adrenergic blockade. Nevertheless the data is compatible with the idea that maximum acceleration, but perhaps not peak velocity, gives similar clinical information to ejection fraction. However, we have to ask can we measure ascending aortic velocity and acceleration non-invasively by the doppler technique?

The first approach to answering this question has been

published by Innes et al (8). We used spectral analysis of pulsed doppler signals which eliminated the low frequency aortic wall components and determined the intensity weighted mean velocity signal. In a test rig, good linear correlations were obtained between peak velocity and maximum acceleration measured by the doppler technique and simultaneously by electromagnetic transducer. However, the linear regression lines did not coincide well with the lines of identity. In patients these variables were correlated simultaneously between the doppler method and the Mills electromagnetic velocity transducer. There was variability between patients as to the excellence of correspondence, but the systematic error of the rig test disappeared and when the data for the whole patient group was pooled, a good overall correlation was obtained. Coincidence was obtained when the integrals of velocity were correlated, confirming that with knowledge of aortic cross sectional area, the method was accurate for measurement of stroke volume and cardiac output. However, as explained above, damaged hearts distend, increase their end diastolic volume and thus maintain stroke volume. Therefore stroke volume and cardiac output are poor indices of ventricular function, especially as the latter is matched mainly to total body metabolic demand.

Another drawback of the doppler method used is that it is somewhat cumbersome for mass use as a clinical instrument. We therefore explored the possibilities of a commercial instrument with very simple operating requirements which is being sold for use in physicians' offices, the Exerdop (Quintin). This instrument uses continuous wave doppler and removes the low frequencies to avoid wall and valve movement artefacts. Unfortunately, we also found that it also removes the whole of the low velocity ejection signals, and that the measurement of velocity integral is therefore unreliable. Discrepancies in velocity and acceleration in the test rig were even more pronounced than with the previous doppler method. However, in the comparison with the Mills probe, when all patient data was pooled, the relationship between peak velocity by Exerdop (PVex) and Mills probe (PVem) recorded simultaneously was:

$$PVex = 2.914 + 0.978(PVem), r = 0.94, SEE = 5.0$$

The relationship between maximum acceleration by Exerdop (MAex) and Mills probe (MAem) recorded simultaneously was:

$$MAex = 1.865 + 0.981(MAem), r = 0.95, SEF = 2.1$$

Thus, this instrument appears to be particularly useful for measurement of maximum acceleration although considerable caution is required about these results. This is because they were obtained by a very experienced user of the instrument with great care to position the transcutaneous doppler probe so that the optimum signal was obtained. In some patients it is not possible to obtain satisfactory signals and the standard output of the instrument, which averages values over a number of beats and rejects data that appears out of line, was not used. The primary signal was recorded on analogue tape and analyzed by computer off-line. More casual usage by a less experienced observer and using the instrument's own print-out may not be so satisfactory as can be seen below.

### DO PEAK VELOCITY AND MAXIMUM ACCELERATION RECORDED BY THE SIMPLE DOPPLER INSTRUMENT GIVE SIMILAR CLINICAL INFORMATION TO EJECTION FRACTION?

It has been claimed that clinically useful information in patients after myocardial infarction can be obtained from maximum acceleration and peak velocity measured by the doppler method (11,12,13). In order to investigate this question we recorded resting supine Exerdop values obtained from the printed output of the instrument and correlated the values with ejection fraction obtained by MUGA. No statistically significant correlations were obtained between peak velocity and ejection fraction or between maximum acceleration and ejection fraction (Fig. 6).

Therefore, we must conclude that under these circumstances the Exerdop method is of little clinical usefulness. However, the two measurements were made on different days, and the patients may have been more anxious on one occasion than the other, leading to variable ventricular function from different adrenergic stimulations. Much more promising results were obtained by other investigators such as Sabbah et al (13), who used the same instrument with simultaneous angiographic measurement of ejection fraction. The relationship between peak velocity by Exerdop (PVex) and ejection fraction (EF) was:

PVex = 0.03 + 0.01(EF), metres/sec, r = 0.77

The relationship between maximum acceleration by Exerdop (MAex) and ejection fraction was :

MAex = -1.72 + 0.28(EF) metres/sec/sec, r = 0.90

This confirms the greater usefulness of maximum acceleration found in our earlier Mills probe studies. It is our intention to pursue this approach further because we know that there is a good correlation between maximum acceleration measured invasively and ejection fraction and we have previously established that the Exerdop can follow maximum acceleration accurately on a beat to beat basis. It is therefore our intention to make ejection fraction and Exerdop measurements on the same day under the conditions of beta-adrenergic blockade.

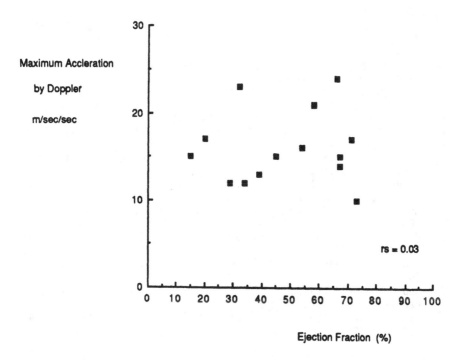

FIGURE 6. Maximum acceleration measured by suprasternal transcutaneous doppler "Exerdop" compared to ejection fraction. Measurements on separate occasions, not under beta-blockade.

## CONCLUSIONS AND RECOMMENDATIONS

For comparing and monitoring overall ventricular mechanical function after myocardial infarction left ventricular ejection fraction is the method of choice. This is most conveniently and non-invasively done by radionuclide counting of the left ventricular blood cavity pool (MUGA scan).

It is possible that refinements of the transcutaneous doppler aortic blood velocity method may make a useful clinical tool in the future. Ventricular mechanical measurements made on exercise remain extremely difficult to evaluate.

For measuring changes in ventricular contractility in response to an intervention in a given individual we recommend invasive measurement of LVdp/dtmax by catheter tip manometer, with the patient under beta-adrenergic blockade and atrial pacing.

## REFERENCES

1. Mills, C.J., Shillingford, J.P. Cardiovasc. Res. 1: 263-273, 1967.
2. Sagawa, K. Circ. Res. 43: 677-687, 1978.
3. Van den Bos, G.C., Elzinga, G., Westerhof, N., Noble, M.I.M. Cardiovasc. Res. 7: 834-848, 1973.
4. Kentish, J.C., ter Keurs, H.E.D.J., Ricciardi, L., et al. Circ. Res. 58: 755-768, 1986.
5. Light, H. Br. Heart J. 38: 433-442, 1976.
6. Bennett, E.D., Barclay, S.A., Davis, A.L., et al. Cardiovasc. Res. 18: 632-638, 1984.
7. Levy, B., Targett, R.C., Bardou, A., McIlroy, M.B. Cardiovasc. Res. 19: 383-393, 1985.
8. Innes, J.A., Mills, C.J., Noble, M.I.M., et al. Cardiovasc. Res. 21: 72-80, 1987.
9. Noble, M.I.M., Trenchard, D., Guz, A. Circ. Res. 19: 139-147, 1966.
10. Bennett, E.D., Else, W., Miller, G.A.H., et al. Clin. Sci. 46: 49-59, 1974.
11. Mehta, N., Bennett, E.D. Amer. J. Cardiol. 57: 1052-1058, 1986.
12. Robson, D.S., Flaxman, J.C., Powell, S.A., et al. Intensive Care Med. 11: 90-94, 1985.
13. Sabbah, H.N., Khaja, F., Brymer, J.F., et al. Circulation 74: 323-329, 1986.

# 7

## STRESS TESTING AFTER ACUTE MYOCARDIAL INFARCTION

Bernard R. Chaitman

St. Louis University Medical Center, Department of Medicine, Division of Cardiology, 1325 S. Grand, St. Louis MP  63104

### INTRODUCTION

The goals of early exercise testing post infarction are to identify "high risk" patients who require further evaluation and more aggressive intervention, to assess functional capacity and provide a basis for physical activity recommendations, and to enhance patient confidence to resume a normal life style.  This review will focus on prognostic considerations of exercise testing in the early post infarction phase.

Patients who are unable to perform an exercise test prior to hospital discharge because of hemodynamic instability, recurrent ischemic cardiac pain, or severe left ventricular failure, have a mortality risk considerably greater than patients who are able to perform a low level exercise test (1-3).  DeBusk et al. reported a six month incidence of reinfarction or cardiac death of 17.7% in 62 patients who had cardiac contraindications to low level exercise testing post infarction versus 9.7% and 3.9% in patients who had a positive or negative exercise ECG respectively on low level exercise testing (1).  Fioretti reported a one year survival of 44% in patients unable to perform predischarge low level bicycle ergometry post infarction compared to 93% one year survival rate among patients who were able to perform the exercise test (2).  Krone et al. reported a one year cardiac mortality of 14% in 192 patients unable to perform a low level exercise test compared to 5% in patients who did (3).  Approximately 50-70% of most consecutive series of post infarct patients who survive to hospital discharge are eligible for a low level exercise test.

## PROGNOSTIC CONSIDERATIONS

The principal factors determining prognosis after myocardial infarction are the extent of myocardial damage, the degree of residual myocardial ischemia, and the propensity for potentially fatal ventricular arrhythmias. The management of patients with acute myocardial infarction has undergone considerable change in the last decade as a result of acute interventions designed to limit myocardial infarct size and as a result of noninvasive risk stratification prior to or within several weeks of hospital discharge to identify patients at high risk of subsequent cardiac events. The risk of post infarction cardiac events can be estimated from the in-hospital clinical course, 24-hour ambulatory electrocardiography, evaluation of left ventricular function from a gated blood pool study or two-dimensional echocardiography study, and assessment of continuing myocardial ischemia post infarction using exercise/stress protocols ± radionuclide procedures within the early weeks following the myocardial infarction. Table 1 illustrates selected variables known to increase cardiac risk post infarction.

**TABLE 1.** Selected Prognostic Risk Factors Post Infarction

| Clinical Course in Hospital | Exercise Testing (± Radionuclides) |
|---|---|
| *Persistent sinus tachycardia<br>*Hypotension<br>*Recurrent chest pain<br>*Congestive heart failure<br>*Recurrent frequent or complex<br> ventricular arrhythmias<br>*Cardiogenic shock | *ST segment depression $\geq$ 2 mm<br>*Ventricular tachycardia<br>*Inability to increase systolic<br> blood pressure $\geq$ 110 mmHg<br>*Unable to complete 4 METs<br>*Reversible thallium defect<br>*Increased thallium lung uptake<br>*Fall in exercise ejection<br> fraction<br>*New wall motion abnormality on<br> exercise MUGA |
| **24 Hour ECG** | **MUGA or 2-D Echo** |
| * $\geq$ 10 PVCs/hour<br>*V tach | *Ejection fraction < 0.40<br>*Large wall motion abnormality |

## PREVALENCE OF EXERCISE INDUCED ABNORMALITIES POST INFARCTION

The frequency with which various abnormalities occur on a low level or submaximal exercise test post infarction are determined in part by patient referral patterns, selection criteria for exercise testing, the level of exercise performed, and the exercise recording procedures (3-9). The prevalance of exercise induced ST segment depression $\geq$ 1 mm, exercise induced angina, and exercise induced premature ventricular beats range from 21-46%, 17-27%, and 15-43% respectively (Table 2). The prevalance of exercise induced ST segment depression $\geq$ 2 mm is as low as 9% in the series reported by Krone et al. (3) and as high as 23% in the series reported by Williams et al. (9). The incidence of complex ventricular arrhythmias defined as $\geq$ 10 premature ventricular contractions per minute, couplets, or ventricular tachycardia is 4-9%. Inability to increase or a fall in systolic blood pressure with progressive exercise occurs in 10-20% of patients in several reported series (3,7,9). Approximately 50-60% of patients will complete the predischarge low level exercise protocol and not have these major exercise induced prognostic markers of adverse outcome.

## EXERCISE INDUCED ST SEGMENT CHANGES

In 1979, Theroux reported the prognostic value of limited treadmill exercise testing post infarction performed prior to hospital discharge in 210 consecutive patients without overt heart failure and free of chest pain for at least four days prior to the test (5). The Naughton Protocol was used and patients were exercised to a maximum of 70% age predicted maximum heart rate or 5 METs. Lead CM5 was the only electrocardiographic lead recorded. In this patient series from the Montreal Heart Institute, the one year mortality rate was 2.1% in patients without ST segment changes and 27% in patients with ST segment changes. Sudden death occurred in 0.7% of patients without ST segment changes and 16% of patients who had ST segment changes. The results of these data have been widely applied in clinical practice and are often used to formulate indications for cardiac catheterization. A follow up study of a similar patient series from the Montreal Heart Institute assessed clinical and

**TABLE 2.** Incidence and Predictive Value of Test Abnormalities During Exercise Testing 1-3 Weeks After Myocardial Infarction

| Study | Patients with abnormality (%) | | | Mean follow-up (mo) | Predictive Value of Variable (%)* | | | | | | | | Events Studied |
|---|---|---|---|---|---|---|---|---|---|---|---|---|---|
| | Angina | ↓ST | PVCs | | Angina | | ↓ST | | PVCs | | Other** | | |
| | | | | | Yes | No | Yes | No | Yes | No | Yes | No | |
| Granath et al., [4] 1976 | 24 | -- | 17 | 24-60 | 33 | 26 | -- | -- | 47 | 24 | 73 | 21 | Death |
| Theroux et al., [5] 1979 | 20 | 30 | 20 | 12 | 16 | 8 | 27 | 2 | 35 | 8 | -- | -- | Death |
| Sami et al., [6] 1979 | -- | 21 | 30 | 19 | -- | -- | 30 | 5 | 12 | 15 | -- | -- | Death, cardiac arrest, RMI |
| Starling et al., [7] 1980 | 27 | 32 | 15 | 11 | 64 | + | 60 | + | 37 | + | 64 | + | Death, MI, UAP |
| Weld et al., [8] 1981 | 21 | 22 | 43 | 12 | 15 | 8 | 13 | 8 | 19 | 4 | 20 | 1 | Death |
| Krone et al., [3] 1985 | 17 | 25 | 43 | 12 | 9 | 4 | 4 | 5 | 13 | 4 | 18 | 3 | Death |
| Williams et al., [9] 1984 | 23 | 46 | 33 | 12 | 9 | 5 | 3 | 8 | 6 | 6 | 9 | 2 | Death |

\* % population that developed an event
\*\* sinus tachycardia (4), inadequate blood pressure response (3,7,9), exercise duration < 6 minutes (8)
+ coronary event rate was 14% when stress test showed no abnormalities
↓ ST = ≥ 0.1 mV ST segment depression; PVC = premature ventricular contractions; RMI = recurrent myocardial infarction; UAP = unstable angina pectoris

exercise test variables predictive of cardiac events in the initial year following the low level exercise test and the subsequent four years (10). Variables predictive of mortality in the first year post infarction such as exercise induced ST segment shifts, failure to increase systolic blood pressure by $\geq$ 10 mmHg, and angina in hospital 48 hours or longer after admission were predictive of mortality after one year. Previous infarction, extent of previous infarction determined by QRS score and ventricular arrhythmias during the test were predictive of mortality after the first year. The data from this study indicates that continuing myocardial ischemia portends the greatest risk for a post infarct patient in the initial year following the event whereas, poor left ventricular function exhibits a continuous risk over the five years of follow up.

The findings from the Montreal Heart Institute confirm and expand the findings of DeBusk et al. (1) who reported a six month cardiac event rate (non-fatal myocardial infarction, cardiac death) of 9.7% in patients who had exercise induced ST segment depression of $\geq$ 2 mm and a peak heartrate $\leq$ 135 beats per minute compared to 3.9% among patients who did not have these findings.

Two studies recently published are at variance with the earlier data (3,9). Williams et al. reported submaximal treadmill test results on 205 patients early after myocardial infarction and found that the only exercise variable that correlated with cardiac mortality was poor exercise tolerance (9). ST segment depression on the predischarge treadmill test did not predict subsequent cardiac events. Krone et al. reported low level exercise test results on 667 patients from the Multicenter Post Infarction Research Group. Exercise induced ST segment depression $\geq$ 1 mm was not associated with cardiac death within one year or with the development of a new reinfarction (3). The ST segment response was predictive of which patients were most likely to require subsequent coronary bypass surgery. Although the data from the more recent studies seem to contradict the earlier reports, the risk of a cardiac event post infarction is increased in patients in whom continuing myocardial ischemia is present and in my opinion, exercise induced ST segment depression, particularly when profound and occurring at low exercise workloads is usually indicative of continuing myocardial ischemia and an adverse outcome.

Exercise induced ST segment elevation in Q wave leads is a common finding during a predischarge exercise test, particularly in patients who have had an anterior wall myocardial infarct. The frequency of this finding decreases over time. When patients who have exercise induced ST segment elevation are compared to those that do not, left ventricular ejection fraction is usually less and the left ventricular contraction abnormality usually greater in the patients who have ST segment elevation compared to those that do not. Occasionally, patients who have exercise induced ST segment elevation predischarge will also have ST segment depression in other leads. The ST segment depression in this type of patient may indicate either continuing myocardial ischemia post infarction or in some patients may simply represent a mirror image response to ST segment elevation in opposing leads. Exercise radionuclide studies will usually clarify this issue.

## EXERCISE INDUCED ANGINA

This occurrence of angina during the test usually predicts which patients will develop angina during the year following infarction, particularly if angina was also present before the infarction (11). This point merits consideration because it often affects rehabilitation and return to work. Not unexpectedly, exercise induced angina also correlates with the late occurrence of ischemic cardiac events. The risk of unstable angina, recurrent infarction, or need for coronary bypass surgery during 11-24 months of follow up is 2-4 fold greater among patients having exercise induced angina than among those who do not (3,7,9,11). The risk of cardiac death has not been shown to be increased in patients with exertional angina on low level exercise testing, presumably because many of these patients undergo cardiac catheterization and subsequent revascularization therapy.

## PEAK EXERCISE WORKLOAD

The ability to complete the low level exercise test post

infarction appears to be one of the best predictors of subsequent cardiac events (3,9,10). In many patients, inability to complete 5 METs of exercise within three weeks of a myocardial infarction is a reflection of myocardial infarct size or an ischemic response. Several studies using multivariate techniques have shown that this parameter is among the most important of predictors of subsequent cardiac events, and has prognostic value independent of exercise induced angina, ischemic ST segment depression and other clinical parameters known to influence prognosis.

## VENTRICULAR ARRHYTHMIAS

The independent predictive value of exercise induced PVC's during early post infarction testing is controversial with some studies showing a significant association between these abnormalities and subsequent mortality or sudden cardiac death whereas other studies do not (3-10). The controversy appears to be related to the definition of ventricular arrhythmias and the sample size necessary to have a reliable estimate. The consensus among many investigators in the field are that complex ventricular arrhythmias ( $\geq$ 10 PVC's per minute, ventricular tachycardia) are predictive of subsequent mortality particularly when associated with severe left ventricular dysfunction. The appearance of complex ventricular arrhythmias during an early exercise test usually indicates that the patient's therapeutic regimen should be revised. The sensitivity of the test for an arrhythmic event is substantially increased when the entire exercise ECG is acquired and computer processed.

## EXERCISE HYPOTENSION

A failure to increase systolic blood pressure with exercise or a fall in systolic blood pressure with progressive exercise is predictive of subsequent cardiac events in many post infarct exercise test series (3,7,9,10). The specificity of this finding for subsequent cardiac events is reduced in patients with hypovolemia and who are taking concomitant cardiac medications which affect blood pressure response such as nitrates, beta blockers, and calcium channel blockers.

## CARDIAC MEDICATIONS AND TESTING

Several studies have shown a significant reduction in mortality in post infarct patients treated with beta adrenergic blocking drugs (12,13). Many patients receive cardioactive medication at the time of hospital discharge which may influence the exercise test response. To examine this issue, Krone et al. examined data from the Multicentre Post Infarction Research Group and compared exercise test results in 107 patients who were taking a beta blocker at the time of low level exercise testing and 459 patients who were not (14). The predictive value of exercise induced ST segment depression, exercise induced angina, and inability to complete Bruce Stage I for cardiac death in the year following infarction was not significantly different in patients who were taking or not taking beta blocker drugs.

## TIMING AND TYPE OF EXERCISE PROTOCOL POST INFARCTION

The majority of low level predischarge exercise tests post infarction are performed using either the Naughton or Modified Bruce Protocol. In general, predischarge exercise tests are carried out to an arbitrarily determined submaximal workload or heart rate response. A 12 lead exercise electrocardiogram recorded during and following the test provides optimal electrocardiographic diagnostic and prognostic information. The test is usually stopped when the patient reaches 5-7 METs, or a heart rate of 130 beats per minute or 70-80% of age predicted maximum heart rate in the absence of marked electrocardiographic changes, angina, or inadequate blood pressure response.

The timing of when an exercise test post infarction should be performed varies among centers. In many hospitals, a low level exercise test is performed before hospital discharge to assess therapeutic regimens, determine functional capacity for exercise prescription at home in the initial weeks post infarction and to determine prognosis. If the patient exhibits adverse prognostic findings, coronary angiography can be performed prior to hospital discharge and a revascularization procedure recommended if clinically indicated. A maximal exercise test is usually performed 6-8 weeks post infarction before the patient returns to work or a full active lifestyle. Another approach, advocated by DeBusk, is to perform the exercise test 3-4 weeks post infarction when the patient has become more active (15). The advantages of this approach are that a greater level of exercise can be performed, the level of exercise can be "symptom limited", and the 6-8 week exercise test usually will not be necessary. Both approaches are reasonable and widely used in clinical practice.

Recently, Topol et al. prospectively performed exercise thallium testing $4+1$ days post infarction in 57 patients with uncomplicated myocardial infarction (16). Only 25% of this highly selected patient population had an abnormal exercise thallium study. Of the 14 patients with an abnormal exercise thallium study, six patients had reinfarction, post infarction angina, heart failure, or ventricular tachycardia in the week following the test. This approach to very early exercise testing in highly selected low risk post infarct patients should not be adapted in clinical practice at the present time until further well controlled studies with much larger patient series are reported.

## EXERCISE TESTING AFTER THROMBOLYTIC THERAPY

Recently, thrombolytic therapy has become almost routine in many hospital settings. Intravenous streptokinase therapy, and more recently selective thrombolytic drugs such as acyl-streptokinase, prourokinase, and tissue plasminogen activator have increased the recanalization rates that can be achieved in the early hours following therapy. The TIMI study has shown that a three hour infusion of 80 mg of double-chain intravenous tissue plasminogen activator administered with six hours of symptoms onset is $1\frac{1}{2}$-2 times as effective as intravenous streptokinase in achieving recanalization of the occluded vessel (17). Larger doses of single-chain tissue plasminogen activator administered earlier after the onset of symptoms and infused over six hours appears to be even more effective in recanalizing the infarct related vessel.

In many patients, a high grade residual stenosis persists after successful thrombolytic therapy, and as many as 15-30% of patients will rethrombose the infarct related artery prior to hospital discharge, more so if the residual lesion is high grade and left untreated. For these reasons, some physicians perform emergency coronary angioplasty of the infarct related vessel in an attempt to improve the recanalization rate and reduce the rethrombosis rate. Several ongoing research protocols will address the issue of whether this strategy of thrombolysis plus emergency PTCA by restoring a greater degree of blood flow to the infarct region significantly improves left ventricular function compared to thrombolytic therapy alone or thrombolytic therapy plus PTCA performed relatively early in the hospital course.

The aim of prognostic risk stratification following thrombolytic therapy is similar to nonthrombolysed post myocardial infarction survivors, i.e. identification of the extent of residual ischemic myocardium, determine the status of left ventricular function at the time of hospital discharge which is perhaps the most important long-term prognostic risk factor, to characterize ventricular arrhythmias, and to identify patient subgroups that may be at increased risk of subsequent cardiac events.

## IS THROMBOLYTIC THERAPY A RISK FACTOR FOR CONTINUING ISCHEMIA POST INFARCTION?

This interesting hypothesis has been examined in several studies. Melin et al. studied 39 patients enrolled in a randomized trial of intracoronary streptokinase and performed thallium-201 scintigraphy at rest before the angiogram and at rest and during stress 5-6 weeks following the infarction (18). The rest thallium defect score before admission compared to 5-6 weeks post infarction decreased by $10 \pm 16\%$ units in the control group, and by $23 \pm 14\%$ units in the streptokinase treated group. The decrease was directly related to recanalization of the infarct related vessel. The change in exercise induced thallium defect score was significantly greater in treated streptokinase patients than in the control group. Furthermore, the perfusion defect during exercise was larger in patients who had residual high grade stenoses than in patients who failed to reperfuse independent of the number of diseased coronary vessels. A submaximal radionuclude exercise cine angiogram was performed 2-3 weeks post infarction in 21 of the patients. The exercise induced increase in ejection fraction compared to rest values was significantly less in patients who had opened vessels compared to those with closed vessels. Thus, the data show that thrombolytic therapy may reduce infarct size by scintigraphic measures, but that exercise induced ischemia is increased, particularly in patients who have a residual high grade coronary obstruction.

Fung et al. examined a small group of 28 patients, half of whom were randomized to emergency PTCA, and the remaining patients to intracoronary streptokinase (19). Successful reperfusion was achieved in 86% of patients in each group. Submaximal exercise thallium SPECT imaging before hospital discharge revealed exercise induced peri-infarction ischemia in 9% of the PTCA group versus 60% of the streptokinase group.

Schaer et al. studied two week low level exercise testing in 19 patients who had patent infarct related vessels at the end of thrombolysis (20). Six patients had an ischemic exercise test characterized by angina and ST segment depression $\geq$ 1 mm from baseline. All six patients had a persistent patent infarct related artery and three of six patients had single-vessel coronary disease. In contrast, of the remaining 13 patients who had a normal low level exercise test, 66% had reoccluded the infarct related vessel and the remaining five had a patent infarct related artery, but no evidence of ischemia.

The clinical implications of the increased prevalence of persistent myocardial ischemia after thrombolytic therapy alone for acute myocardial infarction is illustrated from the results of the Dutch Inter-University Cardiology Study which compared conventional therapy to streptokinase therapy (21). In this study, of 533 patients studied within four hours of symptoms, the incidence of heart failure, ventricular fibrillation, pericarditis, and 14 day mortality was significantly less in the patients who received thrombolytic therapy. However, the incidence of late PTCA/CABG, and nonfatal myocardial reinfarction were significantly greater in the patients who received thrombolytic therapy after a follow-up of 1 month to 4 years.   Nonfatal reinfarction occurred in the same territory as the initial infarct in 11 control patients and in 29 thrombolysis patients.  When the data were correlated to angiographic findings, reinfarction was greater in the patients who had recanalization compared to those patients in whom the infarct related vessel remained occluded.

## CLINICAL IMPLICATIONS

The data from studies of patients with acute myocardial infarction who have undergone thrombolytic therapy suggests that it is indeed possible to limit infarct size if thrombolytic therapy is initiated very early following the onset of symptoms, but that "interruption " of the myocardial infarction may be associated with a continuing risk of potential myocardial ischemia in the infarct related zone.  Thus, the prevalence of ischemic responses seen during noninvasive risk stratification early following the myocardial infarction might be expected to be greater than observed before the era of thrombolytic therapy.  These observations need to be confirmed and expanded by data from other larger clinical trials currently in progress.  It is not clear at the present time whether all patients with acute myocardial infarction require cardiac catheterization and revascularization therapy following thrombolytic therapy.  Certainly, persistent clinical symptoms (Table 1) or a major ischemic response detected by noninvasive risk stratification should dictate early coronary angiography and revascularization therapy if extensive disease or a high grade lesion of the infarct related vessel is found which subserves a large amount of potentially jeopardized myocardium. The role of revascularization therapy after thrombolytic therapy in patients who have a lesser degree of ischemic response (eg. ST segment depression $\geq$ 1 mm in Bruce Stage III at eight week exercise testing) requires further study.  Many such patients will be treated with pharmacologic therapy.  When concomitant myocardial ischemia is noted in the infarct zone and in other vascular distributions at the time of low level exercise testing, these findings would increase the probability of multivessel disease and the threshold for requesting early coronary angiography.

In patients who have undergone PTCA of the infarct related vessel following thrombolytic therapy, coronary anatomy and early ventricular function are known and can be used in the overall evaluation of the patient prior to hospital discharge. In most medical centers where this procedure is performed within 24 hours of symptom onset, only the infarct related vessel is attempted. When the patient has multivessel disease and other vessels are considered for revascularization, the second procedure is usually deferred until the severity of potential residual myocardial ischemia can be assessed at or around the time of hospital discharge. Thus, if PTCA of the infarct related vessel was successfully performed, but concomitant obstructive coronary disease was noted in other vessels, a major ischemic response by noninvasive risk stratification would dictate the need for additional revascularization therapy. If the patient had single-vessel coronary disease, and an ischemic response was seen in the territory of the infarct zone before hospital discharge, restenosis or occlusion of the previously dilated vessel would be suspected.

Unfortunately, many patients do not present to the hospital early enough to receive thrombolytic therapy or have contraindications to its use. As many as 60-70% of these patients will have total occlusion of the infarct related vessel at the time of hospital discharge. The majority of these patients will have a completed infarct and continuing ischemia at a distance or in the peri-infarct zone will for the most part represent multivessel coronary disease. A small number of patients will have early spontaneous recanalization of the infarct related vessel, single-vessel coronary disease, and peri-infarction ischemia.

In most patients who have exercise induced ST segment depression $\geq 1$ mm at relatively low levels of exercise ( $>$ 4 METs), coronary angiography should be considered. Patients without significant electrocardiographic changes able to complete a low level exercise test represent approximately half of the non-thrombolyzed post infarct population. This clinical patient subset has a very low rate of subsequent cardiac events and perhaps are not candiates for early coronary angiography (22).

**REFERENCES**
1. DeBusk, R.F., Kraemer, H.C., Nash, E., et al. Am. J. Cardiol. 52: 1161-1166, 1983.
2. Fioretti, P., Brower, R.W., Simoons, M.L., et al. Am. J. Cardiol. 55: 1313-1318, 1985.
3. Krone, R.J., Gillespie, J.A., Weld, F.M., et al. Circulation 71: 80-89, 1985.
4. Granath, A., Sodermark, T., Winge, T., et al. Br. Heart J. 39: 758-763, 1977.
5. Theroux, P., Waters, D.D., Halphen, C., et al. N. Engl. J. Med. 301: 341-345, 1979.
6. Sami, M., Kraemer, H., DeBusk, R.F. Circulation: 60; 1238-1246, 1979.
7. Starling, M.R., Crawford, M.H., Kennedy, G.T., O'Rourke, R.A. Am. J. Cardiol. 46: 909-914, 1980.
8. Weld, F.M., Chu, K.L., Bigger, J.T., Rolnitzky, L.M. Circulation 64: 306-314, 1981.
9. Williams, W.L., Nair, R.C., Higginson, L.A.J., et al. J. Am. Coll. Cardiol. 4: 477-486, 1984.
10. Waters, D.D., Bosch, X., Bouchard, A., et al. J. Am. Coll. Cardiol. 5: 1-8, 1985.
11. Waters, D.D., Theroux, P., Halphen, C., Mizgala, H.F. Am. J. Med. 66: 991-996, 1979.
12. Beta-Blocker Heart Attack Trial Research Group. J.A.M.A. 247: 1707-1714, 1982.
13. The Norwegian Multicenter Study Group. N. Engl. J. Med. 304: 801-807, 1981.
14. Krone, R.J., Miller, J.P., Gillespie, J.A., Weld, F.M. J. Am. Coll. Cardiol. 3: 577, 1984.
15. DeBusk, R.F., Dennis, C.A. Am. J. Cardiol. 55: 499-500, 1985.
16. Topol, E.J., Juni, J.E., Micklas, J.M., et al. Circulation 74:II-304, 1986.
17. The TIMI Study Group. N. Engl. J. Med. 312: 932-936, 1985.
18. Melin, J.A., DeCoster, P.M., Renkin, J., et al. J. Am. Coll. Cardiol. 56: 705-711, 1985.
19. Fung, A.Y., Lai, P., Juni, J.E., et al. J. Am. Coll. Cardiol. 8: 496-503, 1986.
20. Schaer, D.H., Leiboff, R.H., Wasserman, A.G., et al. Circulation: 72:III-462, 1985.
21. Simoons, M.L., Brand, M., DeZwann, et al. Lancet 2: 578-581, 1985.
22. DeBusk, R.F., Blomqvist, C.G., Kouchoukos, N.T., et al. N. Engl. J. Med. 314: 161-166, 1986.

# 8

## CORONARY ANGIOGRAPHY AFTER MYOCARDIAL INFARCTION

John Horgan

Department of Cardiology, Saint Laurence's Hospital, North Brunswick Street, Dublin 7, Ireland

### INTRODUCTION

Coronary arteriography is the only method presently available which permits accurate definition of the anatomy of the coronary arteries. It permits evaluation of the presence of; a) severity and extent of coronary artery atherosclerosis, b) presence and distribution of coronary collaterals, c) coronary artery diameter, d) the presence or absence of thrombus, e) presence of congenital arterial anomalies, and f) the presence or absence of coronary artery spasm at the time of study.

It is essential in the diagnosis and assessment of the appropriateness and feasibility of various therapeutic modalities, such as thrombolysis, percutaneous coronary angioplasty or coronary artery bypass surgery. It also permits an accurate assessment of the results of these therapies. However, it must be remembered that coronary angiography does not provide information concerning the functional significance of a given coronary lesion. Therefore, while coronary angiography is the standard for assessing coronary artery obstructive disease it is important to realize that there are limitations.

There is a significant degree of inter-observer variability in the interpretation of the degree of coronary artery obstruction. Objective techniques are sometimes used (1-3), and the application of digital subtraction angiography (4) together with automated techniques utilizing computerized border detection or video densitometry have also been used to assess the degree of obstruction.

It has been suggested that the magnitude of obstruction assessed at angiography cannot be substantiated when it is compared to the degree of obstruction found at autopsy. Thus, significant radiological underestimation of the lesions can occur (5,6). However, autopsy studies are not capable of detecting alteration in vessel diameter due to coronary artery spasm and do not take into consideration thrombus which may have undergone spontaneous lysis. Quantitative study of obstructions in coronary arteries when angiography is performed in post mortem specimens with arteries maintained at physiological pressures show good agreement with direct measurements (1). It has been suggested that minimum absolute coronary stenosis diameter correlates best with the functional importance of arterial stenosis (7,8).

## CARDIAC CATHETERIZATION IN THE ACUTE PHASE OF MYOCARDIAL INFARCTION

The management of acute myocardial infarction has undergone considerable change. Accordingly, indications for coronary arteriography and its relationship to the acute phase of myocardial infarction have become controversial and the indications change as more data accrue (Table 1).

**TABLE 1.** Indications for coronary arteriography during the early hospital phase of myocardial infarction

---

1. Acute myocardial infarction less than 4 to 6 hours duration. Candidate for intracoronary thrombolysis + PTCA or CABG.
2. Patient having received intravenous thrombolysis less than 4 to 6 hours after myocardial infarction.
3. Unstable angina during C.C.U. phase of acute infarction.
4. The development of mitral regurgitation or ventricular septal defect.

---

At the present time patients who are admitted to coronary care units of tertiary care centres within 4 to 6 hours after the onset of symptoms of chest pain who demonstrate ECG changes of acute myocardial infarction may be given intravenous thrombolytic therapy. Alternatively, they may be subjected to coronary angiography if they are considered to be suitable candidates for intracoronary thrombolysis, percutaneous transluminal coronary angioplasty (PTCA) or coronary artery bypass surgery (CABG). This aggressive approach is being increasingly utilized and is based on the fact that coronary artery thrombosis has been shown to be present in a large number of patients who undergo coronary angiography early after myocardial infarction (9). It has now been shown that coronary arteriography can be performed safely in such patients (10) and PTCA can be carried out in the setting of acute myocardial infarction.

Such studies have demonstrated that significant stenoses are found at the site of thrombus formation after lysis (11). Also, increasing experience with coronary angiography during this phase of infarction has confirmed that even after successful initial thrombolysis, the incidence of recurrent ischemia and infarction is quite high (12-14). These findings have caused some to advocate the use of angioplasty and bypass surgery in combination with thrombolytic therapy (11). The precise role of this aggressive treatment early in myocardial infarction is not yet clear (15). However, it is recognized that the mortality of patients after acute myocardial infarction is related directly to the degree of left ventricular dysfunction which ensues. The latter is dependent upon the size of the myocardial infarction. Therefore, any strategy which will reduce the size of the myocardial infarction should improve survival.

## ANGIOGRAPHY IN PATIENTS WITH PERSISTENT PAIN

The successful application of thrombolysis requires that patients experiencing myocardial infarction be transported to a tertiary care centre within 4 to 6 hours of the onset of symptoms, and that such a centre be staffed on a 24 hour basis with individuals capable of carrying out cardiac catheterization, coronary angioplasty and/or coronary artery bypass surgery. These requirements create a set of circumstances whereby a regimen based upon emergency coronary angiography followed by acute revascularization may not be feasible for most patients.

However, it has been demonstrated that about 15% of patients who have had an acute myocardial infarction will develop unstable angina within the first week. It is generally agreed that such patients who fail to respond to intensive medical treatment should undergo coronary arteriography with a view to proceeding to angioplasty or bypass graft surgery because the incidence of recurrent myocardial infarction and death in them has been quoted to be as high as 20% (16). Also, such patients have a 25% mortality at three months and 50% at six months (17).

## OTHER INDICATIONS IN THE ACUTE PHASE

Those patients whose clinical picture suggests rupture of the intraventricular septum or the development of acute mitral regurgitation or pseudoaneurysm should undergo cardiac catheterization as experience has shown that surgical intervention in these circumstances leads to a significant improvement in survival (18).

## A NOTE OF CAUTION

It is generally agreed that the risks and complications of coronary artery bypass surgery are significantly higher in patients who have had a recent completed myocardial infarction. It is preferable to permit healing to occur before proceeding to surgery. Therefore, whenever possible, coronary angiography as a prelude to elective bypass surgery or PTCA should be postponed until the convalescent phase. It should be undertaken only when it is thought that the prognosis can be improved by angioplasty or bypass surgery or other corrective surgery. Patients who are convalescing satisfactorily from acute myocardial infarction and who are free of symptoms should not be exposed to the risk of coronary angiography during the early phase after myocardial infarction.

## CARDIAC CATHETERIZATION IN THE CONVALESCENT PHASE

The largest group of patients with acute myocardial infarction to be considered for coronary angiography is that which has entered the convalescent phase (Table 2). It has been demonstrated that there is an increased risk of recurrent infarction and early mortality in patients who continue to experience angina pectoris after their infarction or who have an ischaemic exercise test at a low level of exertion (19,20). A persistently reduced ejection fraction is a significant marker of increased risk, particularly when associated with evidence of left ventricular failure during hospitalization (21). Those patients who have arrhythmias on monitoring associated with a low ejection fraction are also at high risk (22).

Non Q-wave myocardial infarction carries an increased risk of reinfarction and enhanced mortality (23) and, therefore, coronary arteriography appears to be clearly indicated.

**TABLE 2.** Indications for coronary arteriography during the convalescent phase of myocardial infarction.

1. Angina pectoris at rest or with minimal activity.
2. Ischaemia induced at low level exercise testing.
3. Heart failure during the evolving phase of infarction with a persistent reduction in ejection fraction.
4. High grade ventricular arrhythmias with reduced ejection fraction.
5. Non Q-wave myocardial infarction.

It is often suggested that younger patients (e.g. under 35 years) should undergo coronary angiography after myocardial infarction because of the long term morbidity that follows further infarction. However, in young patients with myocardial infarction, the long term morbidity is low as is the yield of multivessel disease after coronary angiography. In this context, the age appears to be unjustified as a precise indication for coronary angiography.

There are numerous strategies which attempt to stratify patients according to the level of risk (25). It is generally agreed that the best prognostic factors are a history of ischaemic heart disease prior to the current infarction, the extent of ventricular dysfunction and the presence of exercise induced ischaemia. It is suggested that these clinical criteria should be considered first when angiography is contemplated in asymptomatic patients under the age of 40 years, even when they plan to return to physically demanding walks of life or remote environments. Careful clinical judgement is needed in those patients where definite indications for angiography are absent.

**REFERENCES**
1. Brown, B.G., Bolson, E., Frimer, M., Dodge, H.T. Circulation 55: 329-337, 1977.
2. Feldman, R.L., Pepine, C.J., Curry, R.C., Conti, C.R. Cathet. Cardiovasc. Diagn. 5: 195-201, 1979.
3. Spears, J.R., Sandor, T., Als, A.V., et al. Circulation 68: 453-461, 1983.
4. Eigler, N., Pfaff, J.M., Whiting, J., et al. Int. J. Cardiol. 10: 3-13, 1986.
5. Grondin, C.M., Dyrda, I., Pasternac, A., et al. Circulation 49: 703-708, 1974.
6. Klocke, F.J. J. Am. Coll. Cardiol. 1: 31-41, 1983.
7. White, C.W., Wright, C.B., Doty, D.B., et al. N. Engl. J. Med. 310: 819-824, 1984.
8. Harrison D.G., White, C.W., Hiratza, L.F., et al. Circulation 69: 1111-1119, 1984.
9. De Wood, M.A., Spores, J., Notske, R., et al. N. Engl. J. Med. 303: 897-902, 1980.
10. Kennedy, J.W., Ritchie, J.L., Davis, K.B., Fritz, J.K. N. Engl. J. Med. 309: 1477-1482, 1983.
11. Serruys, P.W., Wijns, W., van den Brand, M., et al. Br. Heart. J. 50: 257-265, 1983.
12. Harrison, D.G., Ferguson D.W., Collins, S.M., et al. Circulation 69: 991-999, 1984.
13. Simoons, M.L., Serruys, P.W., van den Brand, M., et al. JACC 7: 717-728, 1986.
14. GISSI. The Lancet i: 397-401, 1986.
15. Braunwald, E. Circulation: 71: 1087-1092, 1985.
16. Kellett, M.A., McCabe, C.H., McCormick, J.R., et al. Circulation 68 (Suppl III): 256, 1983.
17. Chaturvedi, N.C., Walsh, M.J., Evans, A., et al. Br. Heart J. 36: 533-535, 1974.
18. Scanlon, P.J., Montoya, A., Johnson, S.A., et al. Circulation: 72 (Suppl II): 185-190, 1985.
19. Théroux, P., Waters, D.D., Halphen C., et al. N. Engl. J. Med. 301: 341-345, 1979.
20. Debusk, R.F., Blomqvist, C.G., Kouchoukos, N.T., et al. N. Engl. J. Med. 314: 161-166, 1986.
21. Greenberg, H., McMaster, P., Dwyer, E.M. Jr. J. Am. Coll. Cardiol. 4: 867-874, 1984.
22. Mukharji, J., Rude, R.E., Poole, W.K., et al. Am. J. Cardiol. 54: 31-36, 1984.
23. Hutter, A.M. Jr., DeSanctis, R.W., Flynn, T., Yeatman, L.A. Am. J. Cardiol. 48: 595-602, 1981.
24. Roubin, G.S., Harris, P.J., Bernstein, L., Kelly, D.T. Circulation 67: 743-749, 1983.
25. Madsen, E.B., Gilpin, E., Henning, H., et al. Am. J. Cardiol. 53: 47-54, 1984.

# 9

# EXERCISE ECHOCARDIOGRAPHY AFTER MYOCARDIAL INFARCTION

Michael H. Crawford

The University of Texas Health Science Center and Audie L. Murphy
Memorial Veterans' Hospital, San Antonio, Texas
Supported in part by the Veterans' Administration

## ABSTRACT

Recent studies have suggested that two-dimensional
echocardiographic imaging before and immediately following low level
treadmill exercise testing in early post-myocardial infarction
patients contributes important prognostic information concerning left
ventricular function.  Studies in our laboratory indicate that it is
comparable to upright bicycle exercise imaging for detecting exercise
induced wall motion abnormalities.  Also, our data and that of others
show that new or worsening wall motion abnormalities after exercise
are highly predictive of future cardiac events and that new areas of
asynergy remote from the infarct location are indicative of multiple
vessel disease.  The success rate for obtaining adequate
two-dimensional echocardiographic images for the evaluation of wall
motion at rest and immediately after exercise is now approximately
90%.  Future directions include the possible addition of Doppler flow
velocity measurements to assess left ventricular performance during
treadmill exercise.  Thus, the addition of echocardiographic studies
before and after standard post-myocardial infarction treadmill
exercise testing is highly feasible and is of considerable value for
detecting resting and exercise abnormalities in left ventricular
function of prognostic value.

## INTRODUCTION

Early post-myocardial infarction patients with reduced left
ventricular global function or persistent myocardial ischemia have a
higher risk of subsequent events.  The former is a potent predictor

of subsequent death and the latter is highly predictive of subsequent unstable angina, infarction and the need for coronary artery bypass surgery or angioplasty (1-5). Both of these poor prognostic features can be detected by cardiac imaging performed at rest and during exercise. Recently, radionuclide techniques have been employed successfully for this purpose (6,7). New exercise induced 201-Thallium imaging myocardial defects indicate ischemia, and reduced lung wash-out of the isotope suggests left ventricular dysfunction (8). Radionuclide angiography can be used to assess global left ventricular function at rest. Also, the presence of decreasing function or new wall motion abnormalities during exercise is indicative of myocardial ischemia (9).

Two-dimensional echocardiography has been used for the quantitative assessment of global and segmental left ventricular performance (10). Also, it has been applied successfully during bicycle exercise for evaluating left ventricular function (11). Recently, two-dimensional echocardiographic imaging before and immediately following treadmill exercise has proven to be highly sensitive and specific for the detection of coronary artery disease by identifying new wall motion abnormalities (12,13). Since treadmill exercise is used routinely in many hospitals for risk stratifying patients early following myocardial infarction, we and others have been interested in applying two-dimensional echocardiographic imaging in this setting. Such an application would accomplish two aims: 1) the measurement of resting global left ventricular function - the best predictor of subsequent mortality; and 2) the assessment of exercise-induced wall motion abnormalities - an excellent indicator of myocardial ischemia and subsequent ischemic events.

## BICYCLE EXERCISE

In order to evaluate the exercise echocardiographic assessment of left ventricular performance early post-myocardial infarction, we evaluated 51 patients prior to hospital discharge (14). Two-dimensional echoes were obtained in the sitting position before, during and immediately after upright bicycle ergometry using techniques described previously (15). Ejection fraction (EF) was measured by Simpson's rule using two orthogonal apical images recorded sequentially during the last minute of each 3-minute exercise stage. We have shown that the reproducibility of left ventricular volumes measured in the same subjects at peak exercise is approximately 10% and EF is 3 or 4% (15). Resting EF was 44+13% (SE) and did not change significantly during exercise (45+10% peak). However, immediately after exercise EF increased to 49+13% (p < .05 vs rest). Qualitative wall motion analysis changed in a corresponding fashion. Wall segments observed to be abnormal at rest were abnormal at peak exercise, but improvement was noted in 41% of abnormal resting segments in recovery (p <.05).

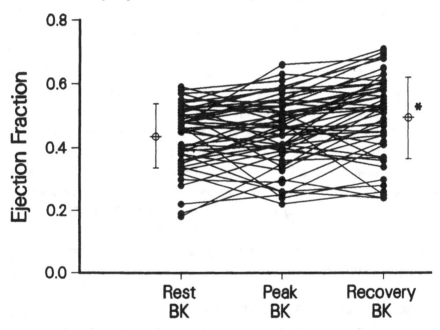

**\*** p<0.05 compared to rest and peak exercise

**FIGURE 1.** Individual two-dimensional echocardiographic ejection fractions at rest (rest BK), at peak exercise (peak BK) and immediately on recovery (recovery BK) of low level symptom limited upright bicycle ergometry. Group means ± standard error displayed as open circles. See text for values.

These data contrast to earlier studies in patients with chronic stable coronary artery disease. In these studies, EF was observed to decrease during exercise and not exceed resting values during recovery (16). However, Dymond and associates have shown that patients with a previous myocardial infarction may increase EF as compared to resting values in the immediate post-exercise recovery period, a response they observed in normal subjects, but not in patients with chronic stable coronary artery disease (17). Also, they found that the failure of EF to rise in recovery was associated with triple vessel disease. Rozanski et al in a large group of patients with stable coronary artery disease noted the same results, but did not divide their patients into subgroups (18). Seaworth and coworkers noted similar results in patients with angina pectoris in whom workload was decreased during exercise (19).

Despite the small mean changes in EF during exercise and recovery in our post-infarction patients, individual bicycle exercise EF responses were varied (Fig. 1). Thirty three percent of patients at peak exercise and on recovery of exercise increased their EF units by greater than 10%, while 20% at peak exercise and 14% on recovery of exercise exhibited a fall in EF units of greater than 10%. Most of our patients had a wall motion abnormality demonstrable on their resting study. A new wall motion abnormality, or substantial worsening of an existing abnormality was seen in 24 of 51 patients (47%) at peak exercise and in 20 of 51 (39%) on recovery. Thus, we postulated that these individual responses may be of prognostic value in the post-infarction patient.

## COMPARISON OF BICYCLE TO TREADMILL EXERCISE

In order to compare the results of immediate post-treadmill exercise imaging to those during and after upright bicycle exercise, we studied 24 uncomplicated post-myocardial infarction patients pre-discharge (20). The two exercise studies were performed within 48 hours of each other in a randomized fashion and the immediate post-treadmill exercise images were recorded in the sitting position to mimic the loading conditions of bicycle exercise. Resting EF (sitting position) was not different on the treadmill and bicycle

**TABLE 1.** Comparison of Echocardiographic Ejection Fraction Response on Recovery of Treadmill Exercise to Peak and Recovery Bicycle Exercise (n = 24)

| Recovery Treadmill | Peak Bicycle* [+] | | Recovery Bicycle | |
|---|---|---|---|---|
| | No Decrease | Decrease | No Decrease | Decrease |
| No Decrease | 16 | 1 | 20 | 0 |
| Decrease | 2 | 2 | 0 | 4 |

\* 3 patients had peak bicycle echocardiograms unsuitable for analysis
[+] p = .08 vs recovery treadmill
  p < .001 vs recovery treadmill

studies (38% vs 40%), nor were the immediate post-exercise values (43% vs 47%). The change from rest to immediate post-treadmill exercise was identical to the change observed from rest to peak bicycle exercise in 18 of the 21 patients in whom this data was available (Table 1). In one patient the post-treadmill EF failed to detect a fall in peak bicycle exercise EF. When recovery bicycle was compared to post-treadmill imaging there was 100% concordance in the EF response (Table 2).

**TABLE 2.** Comparison of Echocardiographic Wall Motion Analysis on Recovery of Treadmill Exercise to Peak and Recovery Bicycle Exercise (n = 14)

| Recovery Treadmill | Peak Bicycle* [+] | | Recovery Bicycle | |
|---|---|---|---|---|
| | No Change | New or Worsened | No Change | New or Worsened |
| No Change | 11 | 3 | 13 | 3 |
| New or Worsened | 1 | 6 | 1 | 7 |

\* 3 patients had peak bicycle echocardiograms unsuitable for analysis
[+] p < .007 vs recovery treadmill
  p  .002 vs recovery treadmill

Also, wall motion abnormalities on recovery from treadmill exercise were predictive of the abnormalities observed at peak bicycle exercise (p < .007), and on recovery from bicycle exercise (p < .002). Thus, we concluded that immediate post-treadmill exercise results are comparable to peak bicycle exercise results.

## PROGNOSTIC VALUE OF RECOVERY LV FUNCTION

Jaarsma et al evaluated 43 patients within three weeks of their first myocardial infarction with pre and immeidately post-exercise treadmill exercise two-dimensional echo imaging (21). All their patients had resting wall motion abnormalities and 18 developed new asynergy not in the infarct area. Of these 18 patients, 17 had multivessel disease on subsequent catheterization as compared to 5 of the 25 with remote asynergy. Thus, the sensitivity was 95%. Mean EF before and after exercise were not significantly different (49 vs 48%) for the group, but the 7 with multivessel disease exhibited a significant decrease from 53+8 to 42+15% (p < .05). Transient remote asynergy also identified 12 of the 16 patients (77%) with recurrent MI or angina during 8 to 16 weeks of follow-up. Therefore, they concluded that immediate post-exercise wall motion abnormalities in areas remote from the infarction identified patients with multivessel disease prone to early ischemic events.

Our total experience with recovery exercise two-dimensional echocardiography post-infarction includes 67 patients with an uncomplicated hospital course who were exercised prior to discharge and followed for a mean of 11 months (22). Clinical characteristics and treadmill electrocardiographic (ECG) findings did not identify the 16 patients (24%) who experienced new cardiac events (3 cardiac deaths, 8 recurrent MI and 6 coronary artery bypass surgery). However, a decrease in recovery EF units of greater than 10% as compared to rest was observed in 7 of these 16 patients (44%) with events compared to 4 of the 51 patients without events (p < .002); and new or worsening wall motion abnormalities on exercise recovery were seen in 10 of the 16 patients (63%) with events, but in only 10 of the 51 patients (20%) without events (p < .001). Although new and worsening wall motion abnormalities were seen in patients who did not suffer a new cardiac event, the distribution of the wall motion abnormalities in these patients appeared to occur primarily in the infarct related areas. By contrast, in patients with a subsequent cardiac event the wall motion abnormalities were predominantly in areas remote from the infarct indicating additional myocardium at risk (Table 3).

**TABLE 3.** Distribution of Exercise Induced Wall Motion Abnormalities on Recovery of Exercise in Relation to Events in the 20 Patients with new or Worsening Wall Motion Abnormalities

|  | WALL MOTION ABNORMALITIES | | | |
|---|---|---|---|---|
|  | New | | Worsening | |
|  | S | D | S | D |
| No event (n=10) | 70% | 30% | 100% | 0% |
| Event (n= 10) | 25% | 75% | 33% | 67% |

D = distance to index infarction; n = number of patients with new or worsening wall motion abnormalities; S = same as index infarction.

Univariate logistic regression analysis of our data identified as predictors of all cardiac events, in order of significance 1) new or worsening wall motion abnormalities on recovery, 2) a decrease in EF units of greater than 10% on recovery, and 3) angina pectoris during exercise. The first two findings also predicted cardiac death and recurrent infarction alone. Stepwise multiple logistic regression identified new or worsening wall motion abnormalities, angina and resting EF as predictors of all events, but only wall motion abnormalities were predictive of death and recurrent infarction alone. Thus, we concluded that a fall in EF and new or worsening wall motion abnormalities on recovery from exercise provide important additional prognostic information to low level treadmill exercise testing in the early post-infarction patient.

Ryan et al also compared treadmill ECG results to immediate post-treadmill exercise echocardiography in 40 convalescing MI patients (23). The development of new wall motion abnormalities on echo had a 95% specificity for predicting a good outcome as compared to 65% for standard treadmill exercise. Also, exercise echo was 80%

sensitive for predicting a poor outcome versus 55% for treadmill testing. In addition, new wall motion abnormalities with exercise seemed to better identify a group with multivessel coronary artery disease.

## NEW DIRECTIONS

Recently Doppler echocardiography has been applied to exercise testing for the measurement of cardiac function. Recordings of aortic flow velocity from a suprasternal transducer position can be readily accomplished during upright or supine bicycle and treadmill exercise (24,25). Using two-dimensional echo imaging to estimate aortic area, aortic flow velocity from Doppler can be used to measure stroke volume. Such measurements have correlated well with Fick measurements (26). Also, this technique has been proven to be highly reproducible (25). In addition to stroke volume, the acceleration of aortic flow velocity has been advocated as a measure of LV performance.

Mehta et al in Great Britain studied 165 patients 3 to 4 weeks post myocardial infarction using aortic Doppler recordings during standard Bruce protocol exercise testing (27). They found that peak aortic velocity, acceleration and the velocity time integral were all lower in those with ECG ST segment depression. In 63 of the 67 with positive ECGs cardiac catheterization was performed. In those patients peak aortic velocity and acceleration were lower in the subgroup with multivessel disease. However, the time to onset of ST depression also was highly predictive of multivessel disease in this select group with positive ECG changes. These investigators concluded that aortic Doppler recordings may be a useful adjunct to exercise testing post-infarction.

## COMPARISON WITH OTHER TECHNIQUES

The major limitation of immediate post-exercise two-dimensional echocardiography is the inabiity to obtain adequate imaging in all patients. Our experience in patients with coronary artery disease is that two-dimensional echoes from the apical transducer position with excellent endocardial identification in two views for the measurement of left ventricular volumes by a Simpson's rule algorithm during exercise can be obtained approximately 75% of the time. Jaarsma et al noted similar results in their post-myocardial infarction patients (79%). However, when only a qualitative appraisal of wall motion abnormalities is required, the success rate is higher; Robertson et al reported 92% and Jaarsma et al reported 88% (13,21). These frequencies include those excluded on the basis of their resting image as well as their exercise image. In our experience, two thirds of the exclusions are based on the resting image and one third on the exercise image. Thus, if resting images are good there is a high likelihood of reasonable exercise images.

Radionuclide techniques usually have a 100% success rate which makes them attractive where this type of testing is readily available. However, echocardiography applied to standard treadmill testing employs resources more commonly found in small community hospitals and clinics. This increased availability of testing equipment would partially offset the problem that not all patients have adequate two-dimensional echo images. Also, if Doppler data proves to be of value in risk stratification, this could compensate for the lack of anatomic information, since aortic Doppler recordings during exercise are feasible in almost everyone.

## CLINICAL IMPLICATIONS

The addition of echocardiographic imaging to routine post-myocardial infarction treadmill exercise testing permits the evaluation of resting left ventricular function and the assessment of exercise induced ischemia. In our experience and those of others, the latter information is of additive value to that obtained from the exercise ECG. Thus, high risk patients with resting left ventricular dysfunction and exercise induced ischemia are readily identified, as are low risk patients without these abnormalities. Knowledge of coronary anatomy is unlikely to be necessary in low risk patients as De Feyter and others have shown (28). Whereas, high risk patients should be referred for cardiac catheterization or put on prophylactic medical therapy.

## REFERENCES

1. Borer, J.S., Rosing, D.R., Miller, R.H., et al. Am. J. Cardiol. 46: 1-12, 1980.
2. Waters, D.D., Bosch, X., Bouchard, A., et al. J. Am. Coll. Cardiol. 5: 1-8, 1985.
3. Starling, M.R., Crawford, M.H., Henry, R.L., et al. Am. J. Cardiol. 57: 532-537, 1986.
4. Starling, M.R., Crawford, M.H., Kennedy, G.T., et al. Am. J. Cardiol. 46: 909-914, 1980.
5. Krone, R.J., Gillespie, J.A., Weld, F.M., et al. Circulation 71: 80-89, 1985.
6. Corbett, J.R., Dehmer, G.J., Lewis S.E., et al. Circulation 64: 535-544, 1981.
7. Hung, J., Goris, M.L., Nash, E., et al. Am. J. Cardiol. 53: 1221-1227, 1984.
8. Gibson, R.S., Watson, D.D., Craddock, G.B., et al. Circulation 68: 321-336, 1983.
9. Nicod P., Corbett, J.R., Firth, B.G., et al. Am. J. Cardiol. 52: 30-36, 1983.
10. Starling, M.R., Crawford, M.H., Sorensen, S.G., et al. Circulation 63: 1075-1084, 1981.
11. Crawford, M.H., Petru, M.A., Amon, K.W., et al. Am. J. Cardiol. 53: 42-46, 1984.
12. Limacher, M.C., Quinones, M.A., Poliner, L.R., et al. Circulation 67: 1211-1218, 1983.
13. Robertson, W.S., Feigenbaum, H., Armstrong, W.F., et al. J. Am. Coll. Cardiol. 2: 1085-1091, 1983.
14. Dell'Italia, L.F., Amon, K.W., Crawford, M.H. J. Am. Coll. Cardiol. 3: 613, 1984 (Abstr).
15. Crawford, M.H., Amon K.W., Vance W.S. Am. J. Cardiol. 51: 1-6, 1983.
16. Okada, R.D., Boucher, C.A., Strauss, H.W., Pohost, G.M. Am. J. Cardiol. 46: 1188-1204, 1980.
17. Dymond, D.S., Foster C., Grenier, R.P., et al. Am. J. Cardiol. 53: 1532-1537, 1984.
18. Rozanski, A., Elkayam, U., Berman, D.S., et al. Circulation 67: 529-535, 1983.
19. Seaworth, J.F., Higginbotham, M.B., Coleman R.E., Cobb, F.R. J. Am. Coll. Cardiol. 2: 522-529, 1983.
20. Applegate, R.J., Miller, J.F., Crawford, M.H. Circulation 72: 449, 1985 (Abstr).
21. Jaarsma, W., Visser, C.A., Funke Kupper, A.J., et al. Am. J. Cardiol. 57: 86-90, 1986.
22. Applegate, R.J., Dell'Italia, L.J., Crawford, M.H. Am. J. Cardiol (In press, July 1987).
23. Ryan, T., Armstrong, W.F., O'Donnell, J.A., Feigenbaum, H. Circulation 74: 12, 1986 (Abstr).
24. Gardin, J.M., Kozlowski, J., Dabestani, A., et al. Am. J. Cardiol. 57: 327-332, 1986.
25. Bryg, R.J., Labovitz, A.J., Mehdirad, A.A., et al. Am. J. Cardiol. 58: 14-19, 1986.
26. Loeppky, J.A., Greene, E.R., Hoekenga, D.E., et al. J. Appl. Physiol. 50: 1173-1182, 1981.

27. Mehta, N., Bennett, D., Mannering, D., et al.  Am. J. Cardiol. 58: 879-884, 1986.
28. De Feyter, P.J., Van Eenige, M.J., Dighton, D.H., et al. Circulation  66: 527-536, 1982.

# III. THERAPEUTIC OPTIONS

# 10

BETA ADRENORECEPTOR BLOCKING DRUGS IN PATIENTS WHO HAVE SUFFERED
ACUTE MYOCARDIAL INFARCTION

Paul. V. Greenwood

Department of Medicine, University of Alberta, Edmonton, Alberta,
Canada

## INTRODUCTION

Since Snow first published a trial in 1965 (1) on the effects
of Propranolol in patients with acute myocardial infarction and
showed a small reduction in mortality, controversy has raged over the
issue of beta blocking drugs in patients following myocardial
infarction. Since then over 20 trials have been published involving
many tens of thousands of patient years, many millions of dollars of
research money, and thousands of hours of physician/investigator
time. Yet inspite of all this effort, we are still uncertain as to
the role that these commonly used drugs have in the management of
patients with acute myocardial infarction in either the acute phase
or the long term phase. Even now, the major basic questions still
remain largely unanswered. These are:

1. Who should receive beta blocking drugs?
2. When should therapy be commenced?
3. How long should therapy be continued for?
4. What is the effect of concomitant treatment with other agents
   such as anti-platelet agents, calcium blocking drugs, nitrates,
   thrombolytic therapy, revascularization?
5. What are the risks, benefits and costs of such treatment?

This review will not be able to provide answers to these
fundamental questions, but will make an attempt to review some of the
literature as to why beta blocking drugs may or may not be of benefit
in the management of patients with acute myocardial infarction and to
ask some pointed questions about the possible relevance of the data

obtained from clinical trials to the management of patients in clinical practice.

## WHY MIGHT BETA BLOCKING DRUGS BE OF VALUE IN PATIENTS WITH ACUTE MYOCARDIAL INFARCTION?

Beta blockers have a variety of properties that might theoretically be of benefit to patients in either the acute phase or the chronic recovery phase of myocardial infarction.

In the acute ischemic phase they might be able to reduce the arrhythmogenic effect of circulating catecholamines (2) and in experimental models, beta blockade or other means of removing sympathetic stimulation to the heart has been associated with a lower incidence of ventricular arrhythmias (3). Prior treatment with beta blockade has also been shown to increase the threshold for ventricular fibrillation in a dog model of acute myocardial infarction (4). There is clinical evidence to support the anti-arrhythmic effect of acute intervention beta blockade. Three large scale double blind placebo controlled studies of early intravenous beta blocking therapy have been conducted (5-7). These trials have also shown a trend to a lower instance of either ventricular fibrillation or other ventricular ectopic activity. In addition, in the MIAMI Study, there was also a lower incidence of supraventricular arrhythmias in beta blocked patients.

A large body of animal evidence exists showing that acute beta blockade given either before or within a few hours of acute coronary occlusion can produce a reduction in the size of the subsequent infarction. The probable mechanism for such an effect is the reduction in myocardial oxygen demand produced by the lowered heart rate, blood pressure and myocardial contractility produced by beta blockade. There may also be an alteration in myocardial substrate metabolism by reducing the lipolytic action of the elevated catecholamines for free fatty acid metabolism is also known to be arrhythmogenic and can increase myocardial oxygen demand (8).

Clinical evidence from the three early intervention studies mentioned would also lend support to a trend to a smaller enzyme peak occurring in patients receiving beta blockers, though there are many problems with equating enzyme peaks to infarct size.

A third possible benefit from beta blockers in the acute phase of myocardial infarction may relate to their known anti-platelet aggregating properties (9) which might result in either a lower incidence of acute coronary occlusion or a lower incidence of reocclusion in the acute phase of infarction.

In the chronic phase of a healed myocardial infarction, beta blockers may also have some theoretical benefits. Firstly, as a major determinant of survival following a myocardial infarction is the size of the infarction suffered, then a patient who has received acute beta blocking therapy may have a smaller infarction than a patient not so treated, resulting in a lower overall risk. However, many of the trials have not employed beta blockade at a time when an impact on the infarct size is possible because beta blockade was started more than 24 hours after the onset of infarction. The long term benefits might therefore include:

1. Chronic lowering of myocardial oxygen demand by reduction in heart rate, blood pressure and myocardial contractility, thus lessening the total ischemic load.
2. Anti-arrhythmic effects of beta blockade.
3. Possible anti-platelet action.

Hjalmarson (10) has argued that the evidence from many of the beta blocker trials would lend support to beta blocking drugs lowering mortality by both lowering the ischemic load and possibly by an anti-arrhythmic effect. However, we should also be aware that the use of beta blockade poses many disadvantages and risks to the patient. In the acute phase of myocardial infarction the clinical course is unpredictable and patients may develop sudden complications which would be contraindications to beta blocking therapy such as heart failure, heart block, bradycardia and hypotension. If beta blockers were widely used and used very early in the acute phase then some patients would certainly face adverse effects from beta blockade as these beta blocking effects would tend to exacerbate the complications that they have developed. In addition, there will always be a small percentage of patients in whom acute exacerbation of airway obstruction develops either because this is unknown or forgotten by the patient, or the physician may fail to ask before using a beta blocking drug.

In the MIAMI Study (6) which probably randomized the lowest risk population of the acute intervention studies, and so therefore might be expected to have the least complications, 95% of patients received the full initial intravenous dose of Metoprolol and 91% received the first oral dose given 15 minutes after the last intravenous injection. There were no significant differences between the groups in relation to the development of asystole, high degrees of AV block, congestive heart failure, cardiogenic shock, or the use of diuretics. However, higher degrees of first degree block, AV block, atropine use, and sympathomimetic agents were found in patients who received Metoprolol. In addition, as might be expected there was a high rate of the development of significant bradycardia (less than 45 beats per minute) and hypotension (less than 90 mm Hg. systolic) in patients given Metoprolol.

The chronic use of beta blocking therapy produces a different spectrum of problems as the time factor alone increases the risk of complications developing. Besides the same short term complications, such as heart block, heart failure, bradycardia and hypotenion which might still develop in these chronic patients as the disease progresses, and the patient is still at risk from other known side effects of beta blocking treatment. These include cold extremities, impotence, lethargy and depression, insomnia, nightmares and chronic elevation of HDL cholesterol (11,12). Thus in theory, we are faced with a series of advantages to using beta blocking agents in acute myocardial infarction but also faced with a series of potential disadvantages.

## EVIDENCE THAT BETA BLOCKERS MAY BE EFFECTIVE IN POST MYOCARDIAL INFARCTION PATIENTS

Over the past 22 years since Snow's first study in 1965 (1), there have been a large number of well intentioned, well organized large scale clinical trials conducted on patients who have been given a variety of beta blocking agents after an acute myocardial infarction. Many of these studies were placebo controlled and the majority were double blind and follow up ranged from 15 days to several years. Inspite of the many thousands of patient years of data which has been accumulated in the literature, we still have no clear consensus on either the general conclusions to be drawn from the data, or how the data can be translated into clinical practice.

In 1981 three major large scale placebo controlled double blind studies were published, all showing a reduction in mortality after acute myocardial infarction. These were the Norwegian Timolol Trial (13), the Goteburg Metoprolol Trial (5), and the American BHAT Trial using propranolol (14). The almost simultaneous arrival of these three trials tended to create a climate of enthusiasm that seems to have dulled the critical senses and made physicians overlook an impressive amount of data that had been previously published or that has been published since 1981 that has failed to support these studies. A certain selection of data seems to have occurred and many eminent authorities accept as fact that beta blocking drugs reduce mortality after acute myocardial infarction. Because these multiple studies have used a variety of different beta blocking agents, and a variety of different randomization times after the onset of infarction, the clinician is somewhat confused as to how to translate this data into clinical practice.

In order to attempt to sort out the evidence a little more easily, it is usual to separate the analysis into those studies where early onset of treatment was commenced, that is less than 24 hours, and those where treatment was started later. This distinction is of vital importance in that the mortality curve of acute myocardial infarction is sharply reducing after the first few hours of the onset of infarction, and so many high risk patients may be excluded from beta blocking treatment either because of the development of complications or death if late entry is used, but these same patients might be included if early entry is used. There is thus a potential for more adverse effects to develop in early use of beta blocking therapy, and for a different population of patients to be randomized to either early or late studies.

## EARLY INTERVENTION STUDIES

Hjalmarson, who is one of the principal investigators of both the 1981 Goteburg Metoprolol Study and the 1985 MIAMI Study, has recently reviewed early intervention studies (10). His review is limited to studies that enrolled over 100 patients and where treatment was commenced within 24 hours of the onset of acute infarction and where the study design was of a double blind placebo controlled nature.

He initially reviewed six early studies which were placebo controlled, performed between 1966 and 1980, none of which included more than 500 patients. In four of these studies there was a trend to a slightly lower mortality in the beta blocking group, while in two of the studies trends were towards a slightly higher mortality in the beta blocking group, but none of these studies had 95% confidence limits which would indicate a benefit from beta blocking therapy. He then further reviewed three later trials, Andersen's study on Alprenolol in 1979 (15), his own study published in 1981 (5), and the Belfast Study published by McIlmoyle in 1982 (16). In only his own study was there a significant benefit on mortality from the use of early intervention with beta blocking therapy. His reasons for dismissing the other studies were that they were of too small of size for a statistically significant effect to be shown. However, it is interesting that he did not include the larger MIAMI Study (6) in this analysis. This study enrolled over 5,700 patients of whom 4,127 were proven to have definite myocardial infarction, and this study failed to show a benefit on 15 day mortality, possibly because the placebo mortality was only 4.9% perhaps indicating an investigator reluctance to randomize higher risk patients as this study involved 17 countries and 104 centers.

Inspite of these limitations, Hjalmarson argues that beta blocking drugs can be safely given to a large percentage of acute myocardial infarction patients (his own estimate would be 80%) and that such therapy would be appropriate based upon his interpretation of the data, inspite of the contradictory evidence from two trials with which he has been associated.

Apart from any effect on mortality there are certain other

advantages from early intervention with beta blocking drugs. The early intervention studies have shown that in the acute phase there is a reduced requirement for analgesics, diuretics, anti-arrhythmic drugs, and digoxin in patients treated with beta blocking therapy. However, there is also an increased instance of bradycardia and hypotension, and use of atropine and sympathomimetic agents. In the Goteburg Metoprolol Study (5) there was a significantly lower incidence of ventricular fibrillation in Metoprolol treated patients but this effect was not shown in the later MIAMI Study (6) or in the ISIS Study (7).

## LATE INTERVENTION STUDIES

The bulk of the literature on the use of beta blocking agents in myocardial infarction is based upon the late intervention with beta blocking therapy. The reasons for this are probably because of its easier organization, fewer ethical difficulties, and easier clinical applicability. However, many of the theoretical advantages of beta blocking drugs might be lost by introducing the drugs at a later stage.

Unfortunately, the results of these trials leaves us still somewhat confused. As has been mentioned earlier, there tends to be enthusiastic acceptance for positive results and a willingness to overlook negative results which don't fit with clinical prejudice. Taylor has recently reviewed this area (17) and points out many errors built into these trials. Firstly he points out the biological problem of the decreasing mortality that occurs over a period of time after an acute myocardial infarction and that this curve is a mean curve composing many subgroups all with differing mortality rates who might be expected to behave differently in relationship to their effect from beta blocking therapy. Other problems include the use of death as an end point, whereas other variables affecting morbidity might be of major clinical importance. There are also problems with the analysis on the intention to treat principal as this poses major problems in translating trial data to clinical relevance where clinicians are only concerned with the management of patients who actually take the drug for a prolonged period of time. Also the concomitant usage of other drugs which may interfere with the analysis of trial data, or the effect in clinical usage are important problems in these trials. He also highlights the important problems of patient selection for the patients entered into clinical trials are only a small proportion of the total number of patients considered. For example, in the MIAMI Study (6), 26,439 patients were entered into the log books as being eligible for inclusion into the trial of whom 20,661 were excluded for a variety of clinical reasons as well as trial related reasons.

In order to obtain statistical significance some investigators have resorted to retrospective subgroup analysis to identify groups of patients in whom benefit was statistically significant. Other investigators or authors have tended to pool data in an attempt to prove a point one way or the other. Finally, Dr. Taylor points out an extremely important and little discussed phenomenon, and that is the widely differing placebo mortalities demonstrated by the various clinical trials. The cumulative mortality rates in the placebo group of four late intervention secondary prevention trials of beta blocking agents, Oxprenolol, Propranolol, Timolol, and Sotolol are all significantly different apart from that between Oxprenolol and Propranolol.

There are 10 late intervention studies using beta blocking agents which have used a double blind comparison with placebo. In 6 of these no significant difference between placebo and drug was shown, but in 4 of these, the BHAT Trial using Propranolol (14), Andersen's Trial using Alprenolol (15), the Multi Centre International Study using Practolol (18), and the Norwegian Timolol Study (13), there was a statistically significant reduction in the death rate seen, and in only the Timolol Study was there a reduction in the instance of non fatal myocardial infarction.

If one restricts the consideration to large scale trials involving over 1000 patients which had a high statistical chance of showing benefit, then only three of these studies, the Practolol Study, the Timolol Study and the BHAT Study, have shown reductions in sudden death rate. In all three of these studies the 95% confidence limits did not overlap zero.

However, other trials using the same drugs in other countries have failed to show similar results. A smaller study using Propanolol in Norway (19) failed to show any evidence of any benefit. A trial involving over 1400 patients and Sotolol published by Julian in 1982 (20) also failed to show a significant benefit from beta blocking therapy and the European Infarct Study with Oxprenolol which was reported in 1984 (21) was terminated after enrollment of 1741 patients because of the absence of a positive benefit. Thus although we have three trials showing a reduction in mortality which is statistically significant, we have difficulties in translating this into clinical practice because of the lack of supporting evidence from other studies. As mentioned above, the widely differing placebo mortalities exhibited in these studies, and the fact that trials only include a small percentage of the patients who are seen in clinical practice.

In addition, Taylor points out the major differences between patients enrolled into trials and patients who present in clinical practice. These include a high preponderance of males in the trial participants, the fact that patients over the age of 70 are excluded, thus biasing the study toward the enrollment of the younger age group, as well as the fact that in many studies high risk patients are excluded from enrollment. Similarly we are lacking any data as to whether the effects of beta blocking therapy are peculiar to any one agent or are a property of the group of beta blockers as a whole. There has not been shown any evidence to suggest a dose response relationship between beta blocking drugs and risk or benefit, and evidence to support when to start beta blocking therapy is also lacking as the trials have randomized patients between 1 and 7 days after the onset of infarction.

Taylor also brings up the equally important point of when to stop therapy as we are uncertain how long the benefit is lasting. There has been a tendency in many of the studies for the survival curves for placebo and treatment groups to run parallel after the initial phase indicating that there may not be continued benefit from beta blocking therapy. Should a continued benefit exist, then one would expect the curves to become increasingly divergent.

So where are we with the evidence that beta blocking therapy is effective in reducing mortality after myocardial infarction? I think this depends upon your own interpretation of the data. At a recent symposium in Europe Dr. R. F. Campbell from the United Kingdom stated as an established fact that beta blocking drugs reduce mortality after acute myocardial infarction (22). The evidence I have presented above would tend to suggest that this "fact" should not be accepted without some major qualifications.

## RISKS, BENEFITS AND ECONOMIC IMPACT OF BETA BLOCKING TREATMENT AFTER MYOCARDIAL INFARCTION

Physicians are notoriously bad at estimating the costs of health care and such analysis is generally best performed by economists. The difficulties of trying to estimate the economic impact of secondary prevention are almost overwhelming. There are problems with translating data from clinical trials into clinical practice for trials concentrate on a small selective population and in clinical practice we try and translate this to the wider population. Secondly, we have to make certain assumptions about the numbers of patients who would receive therapy, the number of patients who would continue on therapy, and in those in whom it will be withdrawn or contraindicated. We also have to make assumptions about the numbers of people who might be able to return to employment and further assumptions are necessary about the costs and frequency of rehospitalizations. For example, if a patient suffers sudden cardiac death and does not require hospital care this is much less expensive than an episode of unstable angina which might require repeated hospitalizations and lead to expensive investigations such as coronary arteriography and might further lead to expensive therapies such as coronary artery bypass surgery or PTCA.

A study performed from Norway recently attempted to analyze the economic impact of secondary prevention using beta blocking therapy upon the Norwegian population (23).

Norway has a population of approximately 4.1 million and approximately 7,500 patients between the ages of 20 and 75 years of age are admitted to hospital each year because of acute myocardial infarction. Of these, approximately 6,400 would be candidates for secondary prevention. Using survival curves the authors presented a model for calculating potential benefits of secondary prevention. They used years of life gained as a measure of outcome of secondary prevention and considered three economic elements in secondary prevention:

a. The use of health services - drug costs were moderate but indirect costs were unknown but probably moderate.

b. Resumed productivity which was estimated to be small.

c. Pensions and other transfers which would increase the public expense.

The net effect of all these was an increase in public expense.

They made the assumption that mortality would be reduced by 25% using beta blockers and it would be appropriate to give therapy to approximately one third of the patients. They estimated that in one third of the patients there would be contraindications to beta blocking therapy or they would develop unacceptable side effects, and in one third of the patients beta blockers would have already been given for therapeutic indications such as angina or hypertension. Thus the remaining third would be given beta blockers solely for the purposes of secondary prevention. For the costs of the drug alone in Norway, they would estimate the cost to be $2.3 million U.S. per year or $675 U.S. for every year of life gained. If treatment were only given for two years, there would probably be a slightly reduced efficacy but the costs would be lower. Their calculations made the annual cost to be $526,000 U.S. per year and $850 U.S. per year of life gained. As a final comparison the authors compared the effects of smoking cessation as a secondary prevention measure. Smoking cessation has been shown to produce a reduction in mortality of approximately 50% following myocardial infarction (24). If only half of the patients are able to give up smoking, then the secondary prevention will reduce recurrent death by 25%, the same extent as beta blocking therapy. However, in patients who stop smoking there are no costs other than the loss of taxation revenue from the purchase of tobacco products. If we were able to convince all males who smoked and suffered a myocardial infarction to cease smoking, this would produce an additional 3.3 years of life per patient. This effect was not limited in time.

It would thus seem that perhaps we should expend more effort on patients who smoke in trying to get them to give up cigarette smoking than to treat them with beta blocking agents, and demonstrates the fact that treatment of patients with myocardial infarction must adopt a multi strategy approach.

The final problem we should consider is that the modern treatment of acute myocardial infarction adopts a variety of strategies which were not available at the time the beta blocking studies were initiated and executed. During this period of time the major strategy in managing patients with acute myocardial infarction was to concentrate on managing the sequelae of infarction. Today, the aggressive approach to acute myocardial infarction includes strategies which are aimed at primarily reducing the size of the ischemic damage. These include early intravenous or intracoronary thrombolysis, immediate or early PTCA, and aggressive surgical approaches to the ischemic myocardium. There is now a greater awareness of the risks of ventricular tachycardia in patients with chronic ischemic heart disease and aggressive approaches to this problem are now standard therapy. In addition, recognition of important prognostic factors such as early post infarction angina, ST segment depression on low level exercise testing, inducible ischemia detected by other means such as echocardiography, radionuclide angiography or thallium scanning in the early post infarction period are all predictors of poor outcome. Thus in many centers it is usual to adopt a risk stratification approach to patients following myocardial infarction.

It is fairly easy to identify a very low risk group of patients in whom the risk of recurrent myocardial infarction or sudden death is in the order of 1% per year. In these patients it is unlikely that any further secondary prevention measures would be of significant value. However, in other patients who are at moderate to high risk of future cardiac events, preventative strategies may well be important. However, we are faced with a variety of options which include the use of drugs such as beta blockers, calcium blockers, anti-platelet agents, anti-coagulants and the role of aggressive revascularization by either PTCA or coronary artery revascularization by surgical technique. Thus the clinician is faced with a myriad of possible scenarios based upon the fact that the population of patients who suffer myocardial infarction are not a homogenous group.

Many of the clinical trials using beta blocking therapies have tended to make the assumption that such patients are a homogenous group and because they were conducted when many of the strategies which are now adopted were not available, they may well have been outdated. Also, because the clinical trials dealt with such a small subset of the total population of patients who suffer myocardial infarction and that this population was further biased by inclusion of younger patients, a preponderance of males over females, and other factors, then translation into the more general population being treated today becomes impossible.

Because we now have such a wide variety of approaches to the patients who suffer acute myocardial infarction we will inevitably have to concentrate on the analysis of small subgroups of such patients to determine if limited strategies will produce significant benefit. For once the complication of concomitant therapy with other agents is included, or one spreads the net to include a non homogenous population, analysis of such data becomes meaningless or else the sample size required is so enormous that no clinical trial could possibly be mounted. It would therefore seem prudent to exercise caution in the widespread adoption of beta blocking therapy as the major secondary prevention approach to patients with acute myocardial infarction as other strategies, some of which can be very expensive such as coronary revascularization or very inexpensive as cessation of smoking, may prove to be more effective.

REFERENCES
1. Snow, P.J.D. Lancet ii: 551-553, 1965.
2. Khan, M.I., Hamilton, J.T., Manning, G.W. Am. J. Cardiol. 30: 832-837, 1972.
3. Ebert, P.A., Vanderbeck, R.B., Allgood, R.J., et al. Cardiovasc. Res. 4: 441-447, 1970.
4. Pratt, C., Lichstein, E. J. Clin. Pharmacol. 22: 335-347, 1982.

5. Hjalmarson, A., Elmfeldt, D., Herlitz, J., et al. Lancet ii: 823-827, 1981.
6. The Miami Trial Research Group. Eur. Heart J. 6: 199-226, 1985.
7. ISIS-1 (First International Study of Infarct Survival) Collaborative Group. Lancet ii: 57-66, 1986.
8. Opie, L.H. Am. Heart J. 100: 531-552, 1980.
9. Frishman, W.H., Weksler, B.B. Effects of beta adrenoreceptor blocking drugs on platelet function in normal subjects and patients with angina pectoris. In: Roskamm, H., Graeke, K.H. (Eds.) Advances in beta blocker therapy: Proceedings of an International Symposium, Amsterdam. Excerpta Medica, p. 164-190, 1980.
10. Hjalmarson, A. Eur. Heart J. 7 (Suppl. B): 35-39, 1986.
11. Taneka, N., Sakaguchi, S., Oshige, K., et al. Metabolism 25: 1071-1075, 1976.
12. Leren, P., Foss, P.O., Helgeland, A., et al. Lancet ii: 4-6, 1980.
13. The Norwegian Multi Centre Study Group. N. Engl. J. Med. 304: 801-807, 1981.
14. Beta Blocker Heart Attack Trial Research Group. JAMA 247: 1707-1714, 1982.
15. Andersen, M.P., Bechsgaard, P., Frederiksen, J., et al. Lancet ii: 865-872, 1979.
16. Boyle, D.M., Barber, J.M., McIlmoyle, L., et al. Br. Heart J. 49: 229-233, 1983.
17. Taylor, S.H. Eur. Heart J. 7 (Suppl. B): 41-49, 1986.
18. Multicentre International Study. Br. Med. J. 2: 419-421, 1977.
19. Hansteen, V., Moinchen, E., Lorentsen, E., et al. Br. Med. J. 1: 1142-1147, 1982.
20. Julian, D.G. Lancet i: 1142-1147, 1982.
21. European Infarction Study Group (EIS). Eur. Heart J. 5: 189-202, 1984.
22. Campbell, R.W.F., Bourke, J. Eur. Heart J. 7 (Suppl. A): 119-121, 1986.
23. Hjart, P.F., Waaler, H. Eur. Heart J. 7 (Suppl. B): 67-73, 1986.
24. Daly, L.E., Mulcahy, R., Graham, I.M., Hickey, N. Br. Med. J. 287: 324-326, 1983.

# 11

## PERCUTANEOUS TRANSLUMINAL CORONARY ANGIOPLASTY AFTER MYOCARDIAL INFARCTION

M.G. Bourassa, P.R. David, R. Bonan, D. O. Williams, R. Holubkov, S.F. Kelsey, K. M. Detre

Montreal Heart Insitute, Montreal, Quebec, Canada, and the NHLBI PTCA Registry, Data Coordinating Center, University of Pittsburg, PA, USA

Significant coronary atherosclerosis has been documented in most patients with acute myocardial infarction (1-4). Although the pathogenesis of myocardial infarction is complex and may involve coronary spasm or ulceration and rupture of the atherosclerotic plaque in some patients (5), a coronary artery thrombus is almost always present and plays a central role in the production of acute ischemia (6). Myocardial necrosis depends on the intensity and location of the ischemia and on collateral blood flow (7). In experimental preparations, irreversible necrosis begins within one-half hour after the coronary occlusion and spreads progressively from the endocardium to the epicardium (8). In patients with acute coronary thrombosis and few pre-existing collateral vessels, myocardial necrosis might evolve rapidly in a pattern which is very similar to that observed following coronary occlusion in dogs. In these patients, reperfusion of the infarct-related artery should be initiated very early in order to reduce infarct size and to preserve some residual left ventricular function. However, in patients with previous collateral vessels or with incomplete or intermittent coronary occlusion, myocardial necrosis may evolve more slowly. Early recanalization of the infarct-related artery would clearly be of greatest benefit to these patients.

Although still an experimental procedure in patients with evolving myocardial infarction, PTCA has been applied in different clinical settings, either alone or in conjunction with intravenous or intracoronary thrombolytic agents such as streptokinase, urokinase and tissue plasminogen activator (9-12). The present report will focus mainly on two important aspects of this new therapeutic option: the optimal timing of PTCA in patients with evolving myocardial infarction, and its potential role in preserving left ventricular function and in improving long term prognosis.

TABLE 1. NHLBI PTCA Registry in 1985. Baseline Clinical and Angiographic Characteristics.

| | Acute or Recent MI (n=114) | | No Acute or Recent MI (n=890) | | Difference between groups p value |
|---|---|---|---|---|---|
| | n | % | n | % | |
| Mean Age | | 56.8 | | 57.4 | NS |
| Elderly (65 & over) | 31 | 27.2 | 242 | 27.2 | NS |
| Males | 89 | 78.1 | 658 | 73.9 | NS |
| Hx Diabetes | 10 | 8.8 | 123 | 14.0 | NS |
| Hx Hypertension | 37 | 33.3 | 401 | 45.7 | <.05 |
| Prior MI | 21 | 18.4 | 343 | 38.5 | <.001 |
| Prior CABG | 4 | 3.5 | 120 | 13.5 | <.01 |
| Hx. Con. Heart Fail. | 11 | 10.3 | 41 | 4.8 | <.05 |
| Inoper./High Risk | 16 | 14.2 | 76 | 8.7 | NS |
| Angina | | | | | <.001 |
| Unstable | 83 | 72.8 | 481 | 54.0 | |
| Stable Class 3,4 | 2 | 1.8 | 162 | 18.2 | |
| Stable Class 1,2 | 8 | 7.0 | 226 | 25.4 | |
| Never had Angina | 18 | 15.8 | 20 | 2.2 | |
| Vessel Disease | | | | | NS |
| Single | 47 | 41.2 | 409 | 46.0 | |
| Double | 45 | 39.5 | 270 | 30.3 | |
| Triple | 20 | 17.5 | 197 | 22.1 | |
| Left Main | 2 | 1.8 | 14 | 1.6 | |
| Eject.Frac. < 50% | | | | | <.001 |
| less than 40% | 12 | 12.8 | 33 | 4.7 | |
| 40-49% | 24 | 25.5 | 99 | 14.2 | |
| 50% and over | 58 | 61.7 | 565 | 81.1 | |

MI: myocardial infarction; CABG: coronary artery bypass grafting

## NHLBI PTCA REGISTRY IN 1985

Among 1004 patients from 16 centers in the United States and Canada enrolled in a NHLBI PTCA Registry between August 1985 and November 1985, 114 patients (11%) received PTCA for a recent myocardial infarction. Table 1 shows the baseline clinical and angiographic characteristics of these 114 patients and compares them with those of the 890 patients in the Registry who underwent PTCA for conventional indications.

## Clinical Characteristics

Patients with and without recent myocardial infarction did not differ in the following characteristics: gender (78.1 vs 73.9% males), elderly patients ( $\geq$ 65 years) (27% in both groups), history of diabetes (8.8 vs 14%), and patients considered inoperable or at high risk for coronary artery bypass grafting (14.2 vs 8.7%)

Significant differences between the two groups were observed in the following clinical parameters: history of hypertension, prior myocardial infarction, prior coronary artery bypass grafting, history of or presence of congestive heart failure, and angina pectoris prior to PTCA. Patients in the recent infarction group had less hypertension (33.3 vs 45.7%, p < .05), fewer prior myocardial infarctions (18.4 vs 38.5, p < .001), fewer prior bypass surgeries (3.5 vs 13.5%, p < .01), but less frequent stable angina (8.8 vs 43.6%, p < .001), and also more frequent absence of chest pain (15.8 vs 2.2%, p < .001) prior to PTCA than patients in the non-infarction group.

## Angiographic Characteristics

The degree of severity of coronary artery disease was similar in both groups. A coronary artery stenosis was considered clinically significant when there was 50% or greater reduction in internal diameter of a major coronary artery. Using this definition, single vessel disease was present in 41.2% of the patients in the recent infarction group and in 46.0% in the non-infarction group. Multivessel disease was present in 57.0% of the patients in the recent infarction group and in 52.4% in the non-infarction group. Finally, left main coronary artery disease was present in 1.8% of the patients in the recent infarction group and in 1.6% in the non-infarction group.

Patients in the recent infarction group had a significantly greater degree of left ventricular dysfunction prior to PTCA (p < .001) than patients in the non-infarction group. Only 61.7% of the patients in the recent infarction group had a normal (50% or greater) ejection fraction, compared with 81.1% in the non-infarction group.

An ejection fraction between 40 and 49% was found in 25.5% of the patients in the recent infarction group versus 14.2% in the non-infarction group and an ejection fraction less than 40% in 12.8% of the patients in the recent infarction group versus 4.7% in the non-infarction group.

Thus, although the extent and severity of coronary artery disease was similar in both groups, patients who underwent PTCA after an acute or recent myocardial infarction had more frequent unstable angina, more frequent congestive heart failure and a greater degree of left ventricular dysfunction than patients who underwent PTCA for more conventional indications.

**TABLE 2.** NHLBI PTCA Registry in 1985. Early Angiographic Success and Major Complications

|  | Acute or Recent MI (n=114) | | No Acute or Recent MI (n=890) | | Difference between groups p value |
|---|---|---|---|---|---|
|  | n | % | n | % |  |
| Some attempted lesions reduced by $\geq$ 20% | 109 | 95.6 | 815 | 91.6 | NS |
| All attempted lesions reduced by $\geq$ 20% | 105 | 92.1 | 730 | 82.0 | <.01 |
| Death | 5 | 4.4 | 6 | 0.7 | <.01 |
| Nonfatal MI | 5 | 4.4 | 32 | 3.6 | NS |
| Emergency CABG | 4 | 3.5 | 26 | 2.9 | NS |
| Death/MI/Emerg. CABG | 14 | 12.3 | 52 | 5.8 | <.01 |
| Elective CABG | 2 | 1.8 | 20 | 2.2 | NS |

MI: myocardial infarction; CABG: coronary artery bypass grafting

Angiographic Success and Major Procedure-Related Complications

As shown in Table 2, the rate of early angiographic success following PTCA in patients with recent or acute myocardial infarction was very high and compared very favorably to that of patients who underwent PTCA for other indications.

In patients with acute or recent infarctions in whom coronary angiography documents a subtotal stenosis of the infarct-related artery, the technique of PTCA is exactly the same as in patients undergoing PTCA for other indications. In patients with an acute or recent occlusion of the infarct-related artery following myocardial infarction, the thrombotic occlusion is usually very soft and is easily crossed by the guidewire which follows the path of least resistance through the occlusion (Figure 1). The course of the vessel can usually be estimated by faint collaterals or by a tapered occlusion.

Table 2 also shows that the combined rate of major procedure related complications, including death, non-fatal myocardial infarction and emergency bypass surgery, was 12.3%, approximately twice as frequent as in patients undergoing routine PTCA. Among these three major events, only mortality was more frequent in the acute or recent infarction group (4.4%) versus 0.7% for patients undergoing PTCA for other indications (p < .01).

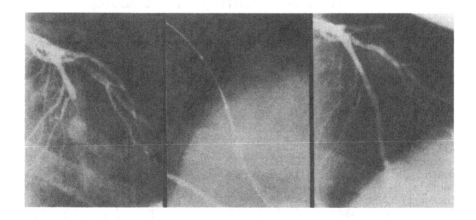

**FIGURE 1.** Cineangiographic pictures taken approximately two hours after onset of an anterior myocardial infarction in a 42 year old male patient. The left anterior descending artery was occluded and there were no visible collaterals distal to the occlusion (left panel). The thrombotic occlusion was easily crossed by the guidewire and a balloon catheter was positioned at the site of the lesion (middle panel). Balloon dilatation resulted in patency of the left anterior descending artery with practically no residual coronary lesion (right panel).

Athough these selected patients are not representative of the
total population of patients hospitalized for an acute or evolving
myocardial infarction, they had several unfavorable prognostic
factors and a hospital mortality rate of 4.4% is probably acceptable
for this high-risk subgroup.

Time from Myocardial Infarction to Onset of PTCA

Table 3 shows early angiographic success and major procedure
related complications in four different subsets of patients defined
by the time interval between the onset of ischemic pain and
revascularization by PTCA.  Thirty patients underwent urgent PTCA,
within six hours after the onset of ischemic pain; 29 had a delayed
PTCA, between 7 and 48 hours after the onset of chest pain; 24 had
PTCA before hospital discharge, between three and ten days after the
onset of pain; and finally, 31 patients had routine PTCA, more than
ten days after the onset of infarction.

**TABLE 3.** NHLBI PTCA Registry in 1985. Angiographic Success and
Major Complications in Different Patient Subgroups.

| Time from MI onset to PTCA | < 6 hrs (n=30) | | 7-48 hrs (n=29) | | > 48 hours to 10 days (n=24) | | > 10 days (n=31) | |
|---|---|---|---|---|---|---|---|---|
| | n | % | n | % | n | % | n | % |
| Thrombolytic therapy | 8 | 26.7 | 15 | 51.7 | | | | |
| Some attempted lesions reduced by ≥ 20% | 29 | 96.7 | 28 | 96.6 | 23 | 95.8 | 29 | 93.5 |
| All attempted lesions reduced by ≥ 20% | 28 | 93.3 | 28 | 96.6 | 23 | 95.8 | 29 | 93.5 |
| Death | 1 | 3.3 | 4 | 13.8 | 0 | 0.0 | 0 | 0.0 |
| Nonfatal MI | 0 | 0.0 | 2 | 6.9 | 3 | 12.5 | 0 | 0.0 |
| Emergency CABG | 3 | 10.0 | 1 | 3.4 | 0 | 0.0 | 0 | 0.0 |
| Death/MI/Emer. CABG | 4 | 13.3 | 7 | 24.1 | 3 | 12.5 | 0 | 0.0 |
| Elective CABG | 0 | 0.0 | 1 | 3.4 | 1 | 4.2 | 0 | 0.0 |

MI: myocardial infarction; CABG; coronary artery bypass grafting
Significance tests were not performed to compare these subgroups.

The rate of early angiographic success was similar in the four
subgroups.  At least one attempted lesion was successfully dilated
(internal diameter of stenosis reduced by 20% or more) in 96.7, 96.6,
95.8 and 93.5% of the patients, respectively.  All attempted lesions

(34, 42, 38 and 48 lesions) were successfully dilated in 93.3, 96.6, 95.8 and 93.5%, respectively. Finally, mean stenosis change of successfully dilated lesions was 62.3, 57.9, 55.0 and 58.8% respectively.

Although these subgroups are relatively small, there appears to be notable differences in the major procedure related complication rates among them. These data can be useful to establish guidelines in the planning of PTCA in patients with acute or evolving myocardial infarction.

Urgent PTCA

Of the 30 patients who underwent PTCA within six hours after the onset of ischemic pain, only eight (26.7%) received thrombolytic therapy before or after PTCA. This subgroup had a rate of major complications of 13.3%, including one death and three patients who required emergency coronary artery bypass grafting for definitive revascularization. Thus urgent PTCA appears to have an acceptable complication rate in patients with acute myocardial infarction.

Whether PTCA can be used alone or should be preceded or followed by intravenous or intracoronary thrombolytic therapy in the majority of patients with acute myocardial infarction remains an unsettled issue (9-12). As stated previously, patency of the infarct-related artery should be restored as promptly as possible after the onset of ischemic pain. Successful PTCA leads to an immediate revascularization of the infarct-related artery and significantly reduces high-grade residual stenoses. With the currently available thrombolytic agents, streptokinase and urokinsase, recanalization of the infarct-related artery is delayed and patency is not restored in 20% to 50% of patients, depending on the route of administration (9-12). These agents induce a generalized fibrinolytic state with the potential for bleeding and their use, therefore, has many contraindications. Our approach may change significantly when highly effective clot-specific thrombolytic agents such as the tissue plasminogen activators become more widely available.

Delayed PTCA

Twenty-nine patients underwent delayed PTCA, within 7 to 48 hours after the onset of ischemic pain. The combined rate of major complications was very high (24.1%) in this subgroup. The rate of procedure related mortality was 13.8%, and four of the five deaths in the series occurred in this subgroup of patients. Two deaths occurred in patients in whom the infarct-related artery could not be dilated. However, two deaths, two subsequent infarctions and one emergency coronary artery bypass grafting occurred in patients with an initially successful PTCA.

PTCA was preceded by thrombolytic therapy, usually by the intravenous route, in approximately half of these patients (51.7%). Failure of thrombolytic therapy may have contributed to the increased risk in this subgroup. In addition, multilesion or multivessel PTCA was performed in approximately half of the patients in this subgroup.

PTCA limited to the infarct-related artery offers little potential for improvement of left ventricular function in these patients. Complex PTCA should probably not be performed during evolving myocardial infarction, especially when there is little time for a thorough evaluation of the clinical situation. Because of increased risk and questionable benefit, the timing of PTCA during this period is not optimal in the majority of patients.

## PTCA Before Hospital Discharge

Twenty-four patients underwent PTCA between three and ten days after infarction, therefore during the same hospitalization as the infarction. Although this may be more convenient for the patient and may avoid a second hospitalization, PTCA and frequently complex PTCA must be performed during the evolving phase of infarction. Patients in this subgroup had a complication rate of 12.5%, consisting of three subsequent myocardial infarctions. This must be contrasted with the absence of complications in patients who underwent routine coronary angioplasty.

## Routine PTCA

Thirty-one patients underwent PTCA more than ten days after the infarction without any complication. At this stage, the risk of the procedure is roughly that of patients who underwent PTCA for the usual indications.

These data suggest that in most patients in whom PTCA is considered after myocardial infarction, the procedure should be performed either acutely for recanalization of the infarct-related artery or as a routine procedure, once the infarct has stabilized, to treat the residual stenosis and additional lesions in patients with multivessel coronary artery disease. In the majority of patients, there is an increased risk and little advantage in performing delayed PTCA during evolving myocardial infarction.

## BENEFITS OF ACUTE PTCA AFTER MYOCARDIAL INFARCTION

Left ventricular function is the most important long term prognostic factor in patients with coronary artery disease (13). Therefore, the goal of thrombolytic therapy and/or PTCA of the infarct-related artery in patients with acute myocardial infarction is to achieve some reduction of infarct size and some preservation of left ventricular function. Although a reduction in hospital mortality has been reported following thrombolytic therapy in some studies (14,15) most reports have failed so far to confirm significant improvement in left ventricular function when thrombolytic therapy is used alone (14-16). On the other hand, successful recanalization with thrombolytic therapy combined with the removal of obstructive coronary lesions by PTCA frequently leads to improved ventricular function (9,11). A recent report by O'Neill et al (12) has shown that PTCA is as effective as intracoronary streptokinase in achieving early coronary reperfusion during evolving myocardial infarction. Residual luminal stenosis in the coronary artery was significantly decreased after PTCA, as compared with streptokinase therapy. A residual stenosis of 70% or more was present in 4% of the PTCA treated patients and in 83% of the streptokinase-treated patients. Increases in both global ejection fraction and regional wall motion were significantly greater for the PTCA group. Thus PTCA is much more effective in alleviating the underlying coronary stenoses and this may result in more effective preservation of ventricular function after therapy. Assessment of long term prognosis and of the risk-benefit ratio of early PTCA during acute myocardial infarction will require additional data, especially from controlled clinical trials.

## LONG TERM BENEFITS OF ROUTINE PTCA

Approximately half of the patients have residual angina and documented myocardial ischemia after myocardial infarction (17). In these patients, PTCA may be indicated to treat angina and myocardial ischemia and hopefully to improve long term prognosis. As a rule, attempts are made to dilate the residual stenosis or recent occlusion in the infarct-related artery as well as additional significant lesions in patients with multivessel disease.

Few long term follow-up data of PTCA are currently available. In the NHLBI PTCA Registry (18), a cohort of 1,390 patients registered beteween 1977 and 1982 from 16 sites have been followed (97%) for an average of 4.3 years. PTCA was initially successful in 892 patients (64%). Post-hospital cumulative mortality in all patients was 4.2% or approximately 1% per year. The rate of post-hospital non-fatal myocardial infarction was approximately 2% per year (8% at 4.3 years). During follow-up in patients with successful PTCA, a second PTCA was performed in 22% of the patients (17% in the first year), and coronary bypass surgery was performed in 15% of the patients (11% in the first year). At the time of follow-up, 70% of patients with a successful PTCA were pain free and 81% of male patients aged less than 60 years who were working prior to PTCA were employed full-time. Thus, relief of angina persists after successful PTCA in these patients followed for an average of 4.3 years. Annual mortality and non-fatal myocardial infarction after PTCA are small. Finally, restenosis of the dilated arteries is relatively frequent, leading to repeat PTCA and coronary artery bypass grafting in 37% of the patients, primarily in the first year of follow-up. The relative merits and cost-effectiveness of medical therapy, PTCA, and coronary artery bypass grafting in different subsets of patients with or without prior myocardial infarction will have to be carefully assessed in controlled clinical trials.

## CONCLUSIONS

PTCA of the infarct-related artery performed within six hours after the onset of acute myocardial infarction has a high rate of angiographic success and an acceptable rate of complications.

Whether reperfusion should be accomplished by PTCA alone or by intracoronary or intravenous thrombolytic therapy followed by PTCA remains controversial. Because a high-grade residual stenosis frequently persists after successful thrombolytic therapy, peri-infarction myocardial ischemia may not be relieved and left ventricular function is usually not improved. Early removal of the residual stenosis appears to be essential for myocardial salvage.

Multilesion and multivessel PTCA should not be performed during the evolving phase of myocardial infarction.

Patients who are seen more than 6-12 hours after the onset of infarction should undergo a complete investigation either at the time of hospital discharge or following hospital discharge and, if indicated clinically, routine PTCA should be attempted on all lesions which are suitable angiographically.

Whether the risk-benefit ratios of early and late PTCA after myocardial infarction will be greater than those of conventional therapy or of coronary artery bypass surgery will have to be determined by carefully designed controlled clinical trials.

**REFERENCES**
1. Bertrand, M.E., Lefebvre, J.M., Laisne, C.L., et al. Am. Heart J. 97: 61-69, 1979.
2. Betriu, A., Castaner, A., Sanz, G.A., et al. Circulation 65: 1099-1105, 1982.
3. DeFeyter, P.J., Van Eenige, M.J., Dighton, D.H., et al. Circulation 66: 527-536, 1982.
4. Bosch, X., Theroux, P., Bourassa, M.G., et al. Coeur
5. Epstein, S.E., Palmeri, S.T. Am. J. Cardiol. 54: 1245-1252, 1984.
6. De Wood, M.A., Spores, J., Notske, R., et al. N. Engl. J. Med. 303: 897-902, 1980.
7. Jennings, R.B., Reimer, K.A. Circulation 68 (Suppl I): I25-I36, 1983.
8. Reimer, K.A., Jennings, R.B. Lab. Invest. 40: 633-644, 1979.
9. Topol, E.J., Weiss, J.L., Brinker, J.A., et al. J. Am. Coll. Cardiol. 6: 426-433, 1985.
10. Prida, X.E., Holland, J.P. Feldman, R.L., et al. Am. J. Cardiol. 57: 1069-1074, 1986.
11. Erbel, R., Pop, T., Henrichs, J., et al. J. Am. Coll. Cardiol. 8: 485-495, 1986.
12. O'Neill, W., Timmis, G.C., Bourdillon, P.D. et al. N. Engl. J. Med. 314: 812-818, 1986.
13. Mock, M.B., Ringqvist, I., Fisher, L.D., et al. Circulation 66: 562-568, 1982.

14. European Cooperative Study Group for Streptokinase Treatment in Acute Myocardial Infarction. N. Engl. J. Med. 301: 797-802, 1979.
15. Kennedy, J.W., Ritchie, J.L., Davis, K.B., Fritz, J.K. N. Engl. J. Med. 309: 1477-1482, 1983.
16. Rentrop, P., Blanke, H., Karsch, K.R., Kaiser, H., et al. Circulation 63: 307-317, 1981.
17. Waters, D.D., Theroux, P., Halphen, C., Mizgala, H.F. Am. J. Med. 66: 991-996, 1979.
18. Kent, K.M., Cowley, M.J., Kelsey, C.F., et al. Circulation 74 (Suppl II): II-280, 1986.

# 12

CURRENT ROLE OF SURGERY IN LONG TERM MANAGEMENT OF PATIENTS AFTER MYOCARDIAL INFARCTION

W. J. Keon and A. Koshal

University of Ottawa Heart Institute, Ottawa, Ontario, Canada

## INTRODUCTION

A variety of surgical procedures may be undertaken during the evolution or resolution of a myocardial infarction.  Early surgical intervention in the first few hours of a myocardial infarction may be required for correction of cardiogenic shock, abolition of life threatening ventricular arrhythmias, improvement of cardiac function in a chronically damaged heart, or replacement of an irreparable heart.  Medical management is undergoing a change from the previous attention to reduction of myocardial oxygen demand, and possible augmenting collateral blood supply to more interest in early reperfusion using intravenous and/or intracoronary thrombolytic agents with or without coronary angioplasty.  Newer drugs give better control of arrhythmias and congestive failure and this has delayed the need for surgical treatment in some patients.

Elective intervention after the acute infarct must also be timed appropriately for the greatest benefit of the patient.  Appropriate elective surgical intervention is the subject of this paper.

## CORONARY ARTERY BYPASS SURGERY

It is obvious that myocardial revascularization cannot revive dead tissue or induce fibrous tissue to contract.  However, in tissue with extensive ischemic damage following infarction there is invariably a mixture of viable myocardial cells and fibrous tissue without clear gross separation of normal and pathological areas (1). The practical problem is that of determining whether or not revascularization in these patients will improve the function of viable tissue.

Selecting patients who are excellent candidates for bypass surgery and in whom the procedure is straight-forward, and easily done with good post-operative results is not difficult. Nor is it difficult to identify those candidates who are poor surgical risks. Those individuals with good ventricles with predominantly localized proximal disease can expect a truly excellent result. The difficulty lies in selecting those patients in the "grey zone" in whom it is difficult to document objective and subjective improvement.

Many surgical candidates with angina post-infarction are treated medically and bypass surgery is held in reserve to be used if medical management fails (2). However, certain serious consequences may occur as a result of inordinate delaying of surgical revascularization including continuing unacceptable chest pain, recurrent infarction, sudden death and the problem of increasing difficulty in rehabilitation because of symptomatic limitations.

Several prognostic indicators have been identified as independent determinants for survival during the first year after myocardial infarction: left ventricular impairment (2-6), residual myocardial ischemia (3,7,8), ventricular arrhythmias (3,5,9) and three vessel disease (6,7,10).

Kaiser (11) in a succinct summary on the CASS trials shows a clear advantage for coronary bypass surgery in patients with left main disease, triple vessel disease, double vessel disease, left ventricular functional impairment or left ventricular aneurysm. Contrary to the initial CASS reports which were somewhat negative towards bypass surgery, further analysis of their results are turning out to be very supportive. For example, in the CASS study subset of high risk patients with three vessel disease and a history of heart failure 91% of the surgically treated patients were free of "sudden death" vs 69% of the medically treated patients. After appropriate statistical analysis to correct for baseline variables surgical treatment had an independent effect on sudden death (p < .001) which was most pronounced in high risk patients.

The appropriate use of selected clinical variables in combination with both invasive and non-invasive testing may enable us to stratify post myocardial infarction patients into various risk categories and therefore prepare an integrated approach to appropriate medical/surgical management of each case (3).

One of the most difficult groups of post MI patients to deal with are those with diffuse distal disease. They are a problem because complete revascularization is not possible. Adjunctive endarterectomy in carefully selected patients may enable some of these to be referred for revascularization. The practice of combining endarterectomy with bypass grafting is not new, however it remains controversial. In two recent papers, one by Kay (12) dealing with a study of right coronary endarterectomy and a second by Qureshi (13) dealing with endarterectomy of the left coronary system mortality was 3.3% and 4.4% respectively versus a mortality of 1% and 1.5% for patients undergoing routine bypass grafting. One-year survival for right-sided endarterectomy was 98% (12) and 93% for endarterectomy of the left side and 80% at 3 and 6 years respectively. A peri-operative infarction rate of 11.9% of the left system is considerably higher than that associated with routine bypass grafting. Patency rates in these vessels are lower than bypass grafts in non endarterectomized vessels, with an early patency in the anterior descending system of 83% (13), in the circumflex system of 75% and with an overall late patency rate of 75%. In the right system (11) patency at one year was 72% in endarterectomized vessels versus 94% in patients with routine grafts. Ninety-four percent of patients receiving left endarterectomies were asymptomatic or had improved symptoms at late follow up (12,13). Kay reports that 76% of patients were asymptomatic after right endarterectomy versus 93% in patients with routine bypass grafts.

Qureshi and his colleagues report on 278 patients undergoing endarterectomy to the left coronary system constituting 28% of all patients undergoing bypass grafting. This is a considerably higher proportion of patients than in most other centers, although they do explain this as being secondary to the fact that no patient at their institution is refused surgery on account of diffuse coronary artery disease. At our own institution we continue to emphasize that endarterectomy is technically demanding and should never be used simply for convenience and that results are not as good after isolated bypass grafting. It is understood that endarterectomy is reserved for patients in whom grafting alone is not feasible.

The future for endarterectomy may lie in the use of lasers rather than conventional techniques. McVicker et al (14) reported a comparative study of endarterectomy techniques in the common femoral arteries of ten mongrel dogs. A comparison of the results following conventional surgical endarterectomy and $CO_2$ laser endarterectomy demonstrated that the $CO_2$ laser presents an attractive alternative form of treatment in this area, but in practice it does not appear to be feasible in the coronary circulation at the present time. The solution however, may lie in the type of laser used.

Farrell (15) has studied the effects of Excimer lasers for the ablation of human atheroma and demonstrated effective ablation producing clean cuts with histologically normal edges, without evidence of either thermal or acoustic damage. The Excimer laser appears to offer significant advantages over its conventional counterparts. Although the $CO_2$ laser may not prove to be appropriate perhaps Excimer lasers with their unique mode of action may hold promise for the future.

## LEFT VENTRICULAR ANEURYSM

After myocardial infarction, impaired cardiac function depends on the degree of distention and the extent of infarcted muscle. The enlargement of the left ventricular cavity results in greater wall tension which is one of the primary determinants of myocardial oxygen consumption. Surgical intervention for correction of congestive failure caused by a left ventricular aneurysm is based on the principal that a smaller ventricular chamber is a more efficient pump and consumes less oxygen. Five variables are important to assess patients undergoing left ventricular aneurysmectomy: size of the infarct (16), location (85% are located anterolaterally and 5-10% are posterior), distention of the infarct area, state of the non-infarcted area and complications of the aneurysm such as arrhythmias, thrombi, and/or papillary muscle dysfunction. Indications for surgical intervention are the presence of a large left ventricular aneurysm in symptomatic patients, particularly with angina pectoris. Appropriate bypassing of coronary artery lesions at the time of aneurysmectomy is recommended.

The operative technique classically described uses cardiopulmonary bypass and trimming the aneurysm edge leaving a small fibrous rim and closing the defect with horizontal mattress sutures over pledgets or long felt strips. However, in cases of large aneurysms such repair results in an abnormal long and narrow left ventricular cavity. Jatene et al have followed Dagget's technique of repairing posterior septal perforations and applied it to anterior ventricular aneurysms. They suggest avoiding septal distention and placing purse string sutures in conjunction with a dacron patch in cases of large aneurysms so as to produce an anatomical repair. In their recent series of 508 cases the mortality was 4.3% and the late mortality had declined. Hospital mortality rates from another series of 334 patients was 8.1% (17). It is thought that the mortality rate decline from 20% to 10% prior to 1977 is attributable to improved myocardial protection, more efficient myocardial revascularization, better protection against thromboemboli and direct surgical measures against intractable ventricular arrhythmias. Late results following aneurysmectomy show a 70% to 75% survival at five and six years and 45% at eight years. These survival rates are better than those with nonsurgical treatment where the three year survival rate is as low as 25% and the five year survival rate is 10% (19).

## VENTRICULAR TACHYARRHYTHMIAS

Most spontaneous recurrent sustained tachyarrhythmias following myocardial infarction are due to re-entry. Ischemia affects both conduction and refractoriness and the electrophysiological basis for re-entry is an unidirectional block, slow conduction over an alternated pathway, and recovery of excitability in a previously refractory pathway in a retrograde manner. Not all patients with myocardial infarction have equal susceptibility to development of recurrent ventricular arrhythmias and morphology and the size of the infarct plays an important role (20). Re-entrant tachycardia usually originates in the peri-ischemic area surrounding an infarction (21).

Medical management can frequently control these life threatening arrhythmias and surgical treatment is indicated only for patients who have failed conventional therapy for ventricular tachyarrhythmias and have reproducible, sustained, re-entrant ventricular tachycardia induced by programmed electrical stimulation. Surgical therapy is also indicated in those patients who develop intolerable side effects to anti-arrhythmic therapy or those who need aortocoronary bypass graft surgery as indicated by coronary anatomy or symptoms of angina pectoris.

The surgical procedure for correcting atrioventricular nodal re-entry arrhythmias has been established. This cryoablation therapy promises to be an effective adjunct in obliterating the aberrant pathway particularly in the posterior septum (22). It also may prove to be more effective in erasing the centers of irritability found in the subendocardium of patients with recurrent ventricular tachycardia and provide a safe alternative to subendocardial resection or encircling cardiotomy both of which have significant failure rates and clinical problems.

Automatic implantable defibrillators are now available and can be used alone or as a supplement to medical and surgical therapy to defibrillate internally and terminate spontaneous episodes of ventricular fibrillation (23).

Patients with recurrent ventricular flutter/fibrillation following a recent myocardial infarction have poor ventricular function with large areas of myocardial infarction or ventricular aneurysm, and significant triple vessel coronary artery disease. Medical management can usually control these arrhythmias, however, when these fail surgical revascularization and aneurysmectomy has been performed. Mundth et al (24) reported 8 patients with three or more than 20 episodes of ventricular fibrillation preoperatively of five survivors of surgery had excellent long term results. Successful outcome has been reported in 60% to 90% of patients who survived surgery. However, 50% or more of these patients have required anti-arrhythmic medications postoperatively (25).

## END-STAGE MYOCARDIAL FAILURE

Cardiac transplantation is now regarded as an efficacious therapeutic procedure applicable to selected patients dying of cardiac disease. Current criteria for transplantation includes patient under 55 years of age with a life expectancy not exceeding 6 months to a year with optimal medical management.

Contraindications to cardiac transplantation include severe pulmonary hypertension, previous malignancy, severe insulin dependent diabetes, uncontrolled systemic sepsis, irreversible secondary organ failure, and lack of compliance. Psychosocial instability is a relative contraindication.

By the end of 1985 over 2,000 cardiac transplants have been performed throughout the world. Most of the cases have been performed using orthotopic technique and a few have been done with heterotopic (piggy-back) technique.

The International Society of Cardiac Transplantation Registry reported an actuarial survival for patients operated in 1985 of 84.5% at 90 days. The major causes of death are acute rejection (26%) and infection (41%) (26). The advent of Cyclosporin has certainly improved the long term results of cardiac transplantation. However, even now the ideal immunosuppression regime is not available and various centres use different combinations of Cyclosporin with steroids and/or antiplymophocyte globulin and Immuran. With careful patient selection and appropriate postoperative care, most patients can now resume a normal lifestyle.

## REFERENCES
1. Ideker, R.E., Behar, V.S., Wagner, G.S., et al. Circulation 57(4): 715, 1978.
2. Hurst, J.W. The perils of waiting. In Update II, The Heart, J.W. Hurst, McGraw Hill Book Co., New York, 1980; 137-140.
3. The Multicentre Postinfarction Research Group N. Engl. J. Med. 309: 331-336, 1983.
4. Fioretti, P., Brower, R.W., Simoons, M.L., et al. JACC 8: 40-49, 1986.
5. Hugenholtz, P.G., Fioretti, P., Simoons, M.L., et al. Can. J. Cardiol. 2: 345-352, 1986.
6. Vigilante, G.J., Weintraub, W.S., Klein, L.W. Am. J. Cardiol. 58: 926-931, 1986.
7. Rahimtoola, S.H. Circulation 72 (Suppl V): V123-V135, 1985.

8. Daly, L.E., Hickey, N., Mulcahy, R., et al. Br. Med. J. 293: 653-656, 1986.
9. Bigger, J.T., Fleiss, J.L., Rolnitzky, L.M., et al. J. Am. CC 58: 1151-1160, 1986.
10. Holmes, D.R., Davis, K.B., Mock, M., et al. Circulation 73: 1254-1263, 1986.
11. Kaiser, G.C. Ann. Thorac. Surg. 42: 3-8, 1986.
12. Kay, P.H., Brooks, N., Magee, P., et al. Br. Heart J. 54: 489-494, 1985.
13. Qureshi, S.A., Halim, M.A., Pillai, R., et al. J. Thorac. Cardiovasc. Surg. 89: 852-859, 1985.
14. McVicker, J.H., Day, A.L., Savage, D.F., et al. Stroke 17(2): 266-270, 1986.
15. Farrell, E.M., Higginson, L.A.J., Nip, W.S., et al. J. Vasc. Surg. 3(2): 284-287, 1986.
16. Jatene, A.D. J. Thorac. Cardiovasc. Surg. 89: 321-331, 1985.
17. Barratt Boyes, B.G., White H.D., Agnew, T.M., et al. J. Thorac. Cardiovasc. Surg. 87: 87, 1984.
18. Codey, D.A., Hellman, G.L. Prog. Cardiovasc. Dis. 11: 222, 1968.
19. Grondin, P., Kretz, J.G., Bicel, O., et al. J. Thorac. Cardiovasc. Surg. 77: 57, 1979.
20. Wetstein, L., Landymore, R.W., Kerr, J.M. Surg. Clin. N. Amer. 65(3): 571-594, 1985.
21. Sherlag, B.J., E-Sherif, N., Hope, R. Circ. Res. 35: 372-383, 1984.
22. Halman, W.L., Ikeshita, M., Lease, J.G., et al. J. Thorac. Cardiovasc. Surg. 91: 826-834, 1986.
23. Mirowski, M., Reid, P.R., Mower, M.M., et al. N. Engl. J. Med. 303: 322-324, 1980.
24. Mundth, E.D., Buckley, M.J., DeSanctis, R.W. J. Thorac. Cardiovasc. Surg. 66: 943, 1973.
25. Tabry, I.F., Geha, A.S., Hammond G.L. Circulation 58.1: 166, 1978.
26. Solis, E., Kaye, M.P The J. of Heart Transplant 15: 1, 1986.

# 13

PSYCHOLOGICAL ASPECTS OF THE TREATMENT OF MYOCARDIAL INFARCTION

Department of Psychiatry, University of Oxford, Oxford, England, U.K.

Psychological aspects of the treatment of myocardial infarction are important in three ways. First, they may help to minimize the psychosocial consequences of a threatening and often disabling condition. Second, they affect compliance with physical care. Third, they may contibute to behavioural changes as a part of secondary prevention. Although, better psychological care is the most obvious way of improving outcome for heart attack patients, clinical practice is haphazard and organized education or rehabilitation is usually only available for a minority. It must be assumed that few of the remainder receive more than simple advice from their own doctors (1).

I believe that not only is psychological and rehabilitation care insufficiently available, but also that what _is_ being done has too great an emphasis on providing inadequately evaluated forms of extra help for patients who are highly motivated and therefore least in need of such help. Aims and methods have, in fact, received remarkably little critical attention. It is often unclear whether the main aim is to restore patients to their normal patterns of everyday life (rehabilitatation proper), or to improve physical fitness or change in risk factors for ischaemic heart disease (secondary prevention). There has been little evaluative research, and what there is, does not clearly support apparently commonsense assumptions about advice, information, exercise or other components of rehabilitation.

Skepticism about the assumptions and claims of much that is written about psychological aspects of infarction should not be seen as a rejection of very considerable clinical achievements, but rather as the most useful and stimulating approach to the further development of any medical advance.

Education and rehabilitation need to be considered critically in the same thorough manner that we all expect for innovations in physical care. We must be clear about aims and then develop methods, which are not only effective, but can be applied to the very large numbers who suffer myocardial infarction. We can best do this by first clearly and precisely defining the psychosocial and social problems that may follow infarction.

## WHAT ARE THE PROBLEMS?

### Acute Hospital Admission

In the early days of intensive care, psychiatric referrals were common and it was often believed that there was a need for regular visits by a liaison psychiatrist. Now that coronary care is routine, psychological problems appear to be fewer. Anxiety, depression, inappropriate behaviour and organic mental states are usually best managed by the nursing staff with support from cardiologists. Families often require more support than patients themselves.

In the later stages of what is normally a brief stay in hospital, denial of distress diminishes and some patients become more overtly distressed. Again, this can usually be managed without specialist help with sympathy, reassurance, discussion and information. Patients and families need, and appear to benefit from, clear advice, particularly if there is the opportunity for discussion.

### Convalescence

Modern active medical management has greatly improved psychosocial outcome, so that many patients are back to full activities within 4 - 6 weeks. Even so, most patients and their families report emotional distress and practical difficulties in the early weeks. These are usually transient but at least a quarter describe persistent "medically unnecessary" psychological and social difficulties (2). Such problems are very varied and not closely related to cardiac impairment. It is essential to be aware that not all the problems described during convalescence should be attributed to the infarct, some may be longstanding.

Psychosocial complications are not only clinically important in themselves, but limit compliance with medical care and may even affect mortality (3). The most important problems are:

Depression Early mild depression usually improves rapidly but is more profound and more persistent in perhaps 10 or 15% of patients. In most cases advice and counselling is all that is required, but severe depression (hopelessness, crying, insomnia, social withdrawal, etc.) requires psychiatric assessment. We find that up to 5% of patients require anti-depressant medication in the year after infarction or coronary artery surgery.

Anxiety Mild anxiety, with or without accompanying depression, is a common feature of recovery from infarction. Sometimes, it is a disabling complication. Worries about the heart and dying, preoccupation with atypical chest pains, hyperventilation and other somatic complaints are very common. Both patients and doctors find it difficult to distinguish between hypochondriacal and cardiac symptoms, especially when the psychological symptoms of anxiety are not prominent.

Work At a time of increasing unemployment, patients have found increasing difficulties in returning to work, difficulties which are worse for those who are at an age when retirement is seen as an alternative. Far too often misunderstandings arise between all those involved, patients, families, employees and doctors.

Leisure Caution about physical activity may lead to undue or inappropriate restriction of hobbies, leisure interests and social life for the whole family. Occasionally the infarct is a welcome excuse for such changes but more commonly there is considerably reduced enjoyment.

Family Concern about a serious illness, anxiety and depression and the practical burden can result in considerable distress and difficulties for relatives. Relationships may suffer and disagreements about the infarction, its treatment and overprotectiveness are frequent.

Sex Sexual difficulties are undoubtedly common but many are not related to the heart disease. Very often they reflect waning interest in later middle life by one or both partners.

Complications of Infarction

Patients suffering uncomplicated infarctions and rapidly mobilized usually make rapid progress without major psychological or social problems (4,5). Those with continuing cardiac problems may be functionally impaired, and in addition are somewhat more likely to describe psychologically determined social handicaps.

Angina Some patients lead full lives despite limited exercise capacity, whilst others are overcautious and inappropriately avoid physical activity (6,7).

Psychological factors are major determinants of the effectiveness both of medical therapy and of coronary artery surgery. Following the latter, the majority of subjects have an excellent overall outcome, feeling less anxious and depressed, leading normal lives without restriction and often substantially increasing their leisure activities. In contrast, up to a third of patients have an unsatisfactory social outcome, not closely related to physical outcome. The social difficulties are very varied and associated with emotional distress and apparently hypochondriacal complaints such as atypical chest pain, breathlessness, and physical restrictions (7,8).

Congestive cardiac failure Emotional distress, especially depression and frustration are common, and moderate and severe failure contributes substantially to the characteristic symptoms of fatigue and breathlessness. We found in series of 120 patients in a recent controlled clinical trial of drug therapy that psychological problems and psychosocial handicaps were not closely associated with any measure of impaired cardiac function or physical capacity.

Pacemakers Pacemakers undoubtedly transform the quality of life of many cardiac patients, young and old. It is probable that such benefits have been undervalued by doctors. It is also true that some patients have difficulties in adjustment and fail to obtain optimal benefits.

Secondary Prevention of Ischaemic Heart Disease

Returning to a full life after an infarct or surgery often

means a return of habits which are risk factors for further cardiac morbidity: smoking, poor diet, lack of exercise and stress. Enthusiasm for secondary prevention programmes has overshadowed considerable evidence that many other patients, who have received no more than simple advice, make major changes in their lives. We find that after an infarct, half the smokers stop completely, more than half of those advised to modify their diet do so, and others increase physical activity and reduce stress. Similarly, impressive changes are seen in the control groups for trials of beta-blockers, exercise training and other forms of intervention.

Prediction and Identification

Analysis of predictors of outcome has concentrated on employment but we need to examine prediction of a much wider view of quality of life. Some patients who are at risk of long-term psychological and social difficulties can be recognized during their initial hospital admission, but is is more accurate and clinically simpler to concentrate on early detection in early convalescence (8).

**Table 1.** Factors Predicting Psychosocial Problems After Coronary Artery Surgery

| | | |
|---|---|---|
| Factors in the history | a) | Previous difficulty in dealing with stress (e.g. history of psychiatric consultation) |
| | b) | Longstanding social problems (work, leisure, family) |
| Preoperative assessment | a) | Moderate or severe emotional distress |
| | b) | Overcautious response to symptoms |
| | c) | Overcautious or unrealistic expectations |
| Early signs of problems | a) | Anxiety or depression |
| | b) | Overcautious expectations |
| | c) | Slowness and difficulty in returning to activities (work, leisure and social activities, sex) |
| | d) | Over-protective family |
| Physical problems | a) | Persistent angina |
| | b) | Neuropsychological complications |
| | c) | Other cardiac problems |

The main predictors of quality of life after infarction are cardiac status, psychological status and coping abilities and previous social adjustment. Predictors of outcome after coronary artery surgery are very similar and are listed in Table 1.

Conclusions

Temporary distress following infarction and cardiac surgery is usual for most patients and most families. Most make excellent and rapid recoveries, even without planned rehabilitation, but a minority suffer persistent medically "unnecessary" handicaps. Problems are more diverse than often recognized, and it is essential both to consider all areas of 'quality of life' and to take account of the subjective satisfaction of patients and families. Crude figures of return to work, sexual performance or other aspects have little value if we fail to discover the individual meaning of changes.

Difficulties are particularly common after complicated infarcts and it is apparent that many people fail to obtain maximum benefit from medical and surgical treatment for psychological reasons. Unnecessary handicaps are also especially likely in those with histories of previous psychological problems, poor coping with stress and social problems.

Description of the difficulties following infarction indicate three priorities for rehabilitation:

(1) Routine help for all patients and their families to enable them to cope with distress and practical problems and make the maximum use of medical and surgical therapy.

(2) Early detection and treatment of the varied and persistent "medically unnecessary" effects on "quality of life" described by 25 to 30% of patients.

(3) A 'preventive' programme that is without great hazard, expense or inconvenience (9) for those with ischaemic heart disease. This means stopping smoking, exercise training, stress reduction, weight loss alongside the medical components of multiple risk factor reduction such as the control of hypertension, beta blockers and control of lipid levels.

## REHABILITATION METHODS

The aims of many current rehabilitation programmes implicity recognize the priorities I have outlined (see Table 2). However in practice the greatest efforts are devoted to the best motivated patients and to secondary prevention rather than true rehabilitation.

Some cardiac units provide impressive, flexible and comprehensive post-infarction care (10) beginning as soon as the patient is admitted to hospital. It is more usual for specialist rehabilitation to have a rigid format, often separate from any continuing cardiological care (11), and to concentrate on exercise to improve the physical fitness and morale of 'low risk' patients. Such programmes take little account of the wide range of individual problems and needs described earlier.

**Table 2.** Aims of Rehabilitation

---

Rehabilitation Proper
a) Minimize immediate distress to patient and family
b) Enable rapid return to normal everday life:  Work
                                                 Leisure
                                                 Social
                                                 Family
                                                 Sex
c) Continuing help for the physically impaired and those needing continuing medical care.

Secondary Prevention
a) Encourage physical fitness
b) Promote healthy lifestyle:  diet, not smoking
c) Reduce stress

Even though enthusiasm is considerably more conspicuous than self-criticism, there have been recent signs of more open minded approaches: awareness that improved quality of life may be a more appropriate aim than secondary prevention, less concentration on return to work as a measure of outcome and greater concern with those who are poor attenders, the elderly and those with cardiac complications (11).

Although "those who run rehabilitation programmes are usually highly enthusiastic and have a strong impression of benefits" (12) there is little convincing evidence (4,11). Far too often it is assumed that apparently common sense treatments such as exercise or advice, are effective, even though this is not supported by evidence on cardiac rehabilitation or on the management of other disabling illnesses.

Most published accounts of the benefits of rehabilitation are based on clinical experience with articulate volunteers and there have been only a handful of controlled trials, few of which come near to the standards we require in the evaluation of post-infarct medical and surgical care (13). There have been few attempts to study representative patient groups, or to use standardised measures of outcome of the major aspects of quality of life discussed above, as well as for cardiac morbidity or mortality.

Exercise

Exercise has been by far the most popular component of both early and late rehabilitation and it is claimed to improve physical fitness and have wider benefits. Early exercise after myocardial infarction has modest training benefits. Although very popular with many patients and therapists it has disappointingly little effect on mental state or any measure of quality of life (4). It seems that well motivated patients enjoy training but do not need it, whilst those who are most at risk of problems either fail to attend or do not find standard programmes helpful. A major programme with "low risk" patients has shown that supervised exercise is no more effective than home based exercise and has little advantage over prescription based on a single exercise test. It is clear that most low risk patients can be satisfactorily treated by systematic advice and exercise prescription, although individual extra help is required by a minority with special problems (14).

All major controlled trials of late long term exercise training have reported high dropout rates and increased physical activity by many control subjects. Despite all the difficulties of interpretation, it is reasonable to conclude that exercise is valuable as secondary prevention for enthusiastic subjects. It is also widely stated that exercise has considerable psychological benefits which by themselves justify its use. However, the only controlled trial to have included psychological outcome measures

found no overall differences between exercise and control groups
(15).

It is unfortunate that most term exercise programmes exclude
both the elderly and those with chronic cardiac impairments. These
large groups have particular difficulty in knowing how much exertion
is possible or appropriate and it is probable that careful exercise
testing and supervised exercise programmes would be important
components of management.

Education

The need for information and advice is obvious but it is not
clear what are the best methods. Trials have shown no more than
modest benefits for pre-discharge and out-patient education
programmes in terms of rather varied criteria. There are major
problems, problems which have been examined more thoroughly in other
major illnesses, such as diabetes, (16) cancer and preparation for
surgery (17). Education is too often a didactic presentation of what
doctors believe is important, rather than a discussion which takes
account of patients' particular interests and needs (18), families
are ignored and written information is badly presented and over
complex.

In the clinical management of infarct patients, there is
usually insufficient recognition of the established principles of
effective communication: repetition and consistency, discussion with
patients and families, clear written information, an emphasis on
general principles of "coping" with a gradual increase in activities
during convalescence, rather than didactic and inflexible
instructions and close co-ordination with medical care. Wenger (19)
has usefully pointed out that new technologies offer considerable
scope for better and more more flexible education.

Psychological Interventions

Apart from basic techniques of support, encouragement and
reassurance, various specific psychological interventions have been
recommended. It is probable that they have common features, such as
education, encouraging physical activity, anxiety management and
support. Their benefits after myocardial infarction are "at best
modest and there seems little reason to offer such help routinely"

(20), although each may be effective with carefully chosen subgroups.

Group treatments   Group treatments are most satisfactory when they combine discussion and education.   They are often not very popular with patients and have not been shown to be any more effective than other psychological interventions.   A minority of motivated patients appear to enjoy groups and benefit (21).   Group discussion can sometimes increase anxiety and uncertainty.

Counselling   The results of studies of in hospital and post discharge counselling parallel those of other methods of rehabilition, modest benefits and some suggestion that the majority have little need of extra help (20).   Sexual counselling is helpful to some, although not all those thought to have 'problems' are dissatisfied or want help.

Behavioural   Anxiety (stress) management and cognitive techniques are now widely used in medicine and psychiatry and could have a larger role for overcautious anxiety patients and the common problems of atypical chest pain and hyperventilation.   There have been no systematic trials, although in a just completed controlled trial we have found that behavioural treatment of chest pain in patients with ischaemic heart disease can be highly effective.

There are also promising reports that a very intensive programme combining education, behavioural advice and group discussion can modify behaviour and reduce cardiac morbidity (22). We need to know whether these findings can be replicated using methods that would be feasible in ordinary clinical practice.

Psychotropic medication   Benzodiazepines are useful for short periods of stress but should not be used for more than a few weeks. A small minority benefit from anti-depressant therapy, although these must be used with care following infarction and in those with abnormalities of rhythm.

## THE ORGANIZATION OF CARE

Review of rehabilitation methods shows that a variety of treatment methods, of which exercise and education are the most popular, reduce early distress, increase satisfaction and encourage a rapid return to normal activities after infarction.   These are important benefits, but it is disappointing that the very few controlled trials have found that such methods have few longer term physiological and other benefits. None of the widely used methods have been shown to be effective or popular with the 25 to 30% who are most 'at risk' of persistent problems.

**Table 3.** Organization of Care

| | | |
|---|---|---|
| A. Routine Care | Hospital: | Identify special problems<br>Information and advice<br>  (oral and written)<br>Opportunity for discussion<br>  (patient and family) |
| | Follow up: | Review of progress<br>Repetition of advice<br>Exercise testing and<br>  prescription<br>Answer questions |
| B. Selective Rehabilitation | | Counselling<br>Exercise training (individual<br>  unsupervised or group)<br>Practical help (work,<br>  accommodation etc.)<br>Behavioural advice (anxiety<br>  management)<br>Antidepressants for severe<br>  depression<br>Day or inpatient rehabilitation<br>Specialist sex therapy |
| C. Selective Secondary Prevention | | Exercise programmes (individual<br>  unsupervised or group)<br>Smoking clinics<br>Weight and diet groups<br>Stress reduction programmes |

I believe there is now consistent evidence that standard and apparently common sense specialist rehabilitation programmes are unnecessary for the majority of patients and too rigid for the important minority who do need help. Many of these "problem" patients could best be helped by more flexible rehabilitation using individually planned combinations of methods. Even so, we may have to accept that a small number, especially those with longstanding psychosocial problems, will be unable to make successful use of any form of rehabilitation.

If we are to provide flexible selective care for all infarct patients, we need a clear system which offers good simple routine care for everyone and individually planned extra help for a minority who really need it (Table 3). The ways in which this is done will depend on local resources and systems of health care. Few cardiac units have resources to provide elaborate care for the very large numbers of cardiac patients, but much can be achieved by well organized care which ensures simple, clear, consistent advice and makes the maximum use of inexpensive aids.

Routine care   Well written booklets and audio-visual methods are useful, but every family should also have the opportunity for discussion of individual advice.   Early exercise testing is useful both to boost confidence and allow detailed prescription of everyday physical activity.   The patient, relatives and all those involved need copies of the agreed plans.   New technology offers enormous scope for improving record keeping and assessment as well as for education (19).

Discussion of plans should be as informal as possible.   For instance, many patients who are reluctant to raise their worries with doctors during consultations are able to talk to nurses or physiotherapists during exercise or education classes.   Indeed, it may be one of the main advantages of exercise groups that they allow the opportunity for patients and families to talk to one another and to therapists in a relatively relaxed setting.

It is often extremely helpful if a doctor or a member of the rehabilitation team has direct contact with the patients' employers to discuss the patient's medical state and the demands of the work.

Selective extra treatment   This requires the same combination of detailed assessment and individual treatment as cardiological management (14).   Successful identification requires systematic review and we find that this is best done by seeing husbands and wives together.   In large cardiac clinics, some time could be saved by using self-report questionnaires in the waiting room.   However, our experience supports the finding (23) that interview by a therapist or technician is superior to self report in the identification of depression. For an adequately comprehensive assessment there is no substitute for an interview that covers all the important areas:

Review at follow-up

Cardiological assessment

Atypical chest pains and somatic symptoms

Physical and social activities: ? progressive increase

Compliance with medical advice: medication, diet,
    smoking, activity

Work: plans and difficulties

Sex

Family: attitude to convalescence

Driving

Any problems?

Enquiry about these areas need not be time consuming. Questions can be asked informally whilst examining the patient and will be particularly straightforward if the medical notes contain clear and brief summaries of premorbid adjustment and activities and of any subsequent problems or uncertainties. It is, of course, necessary to spend some extra time dealing with difficulties that are identified. It is all too common for difficulties to be noted during follow-up appointments but not treated.

We have seen that standard all purpose programmes of rehabilitation are not very effective and satisfactory individual care requires access to the whole range of rehabilitation procedures. It is, however, possible to outline some general principles.

(a) Since many of the 'problem' patients also have cardiac complications, medical and rehabilitation care should be co-ordinated.

(b) Advice should follow general behavioural principles. It should be clear, discussed and agreed with patients and have realistic short term and long term goals. This includes detailed exercise prescription, step-by-step and long term aims and sometimes keeping a daily diary of progress and problems.

(c) Exercise testing and training are valuable but should be used as part of an overall rehabilitation plan. Home-based exercise may be more effective than standard hospital programmes.

(d) Relatives should be involved, both that they can provide support and motivation also to relieve the anxieties and prevent over-protection.

Table 3 lists some kinds of specialist treatment that need to be available after infarction. Anxiety and depression usually improve with counselling, encouragement and explanation, but 2 to 5% of patients need antidepressant medication and 5 to 10% need specialist anxiety treatment. Organized work evaluation and advice can reduce occupational disability (24). Most sexual problems respond to simple discussion and advice, and only a few couples require specialist treatment. A very very few patients require day patient or inpatient rehabilitation.

Rehabilitation concentrates on the problems associated with the heart disease but we have seen that some of the difficulties attributed to heart disease are unrelated and of long standing. We cannot expect to be as successful with such problems but the crisis of a serious illness can be particularly good opportunity for change, since many patients review their lives and ambitions and become more appreciative of family life. The sensitive doctor will encourage them to turn good intentions into constructive changes.

Secondary prevention Advice about secondary prevention should begin early after infarction and progress should be reviewed during convalescence. If the resources are available, extra help should be available for those who can be encouraged to make use of them. Rehabilitation programmes can make a useful contribution to multiple risk factor reduction in promoting stopping smoking, stress reduction and regular exercise. The precise role of long term exercise training remains uncertain, but it may have considerable physical and psychological advantages for a sub-group of enthusiastic subjects.

## CONCLUSION

At present cardiac rehabilitation is haphazard and we need to clarify aims and methods so as to make care available to all who need it. Any substantial increase in availability must depend on making the maximum use of simple and cheap methods. Much can be done by good organization, the use of written information and cooperation with self-help groups, it is probable that even with limited resources selective care can be highly cost effective in reducing morbidity and continuing use of medical services.

There is little prospect that such improved rehabilitation in hospitals or health centres will diminish the importance of care by patient's own physicians. The evidence reviewed suggests that if they are well-informed they will be able to do much to rehabilitate and promote healthier living. However, they need access to specialist assessment and treatment services for a proportion of patients.

Psychological care cannot be separated more than other aspects of management. It should not be seen as a specialist responsibility, even though a proportion of patients will require assessment for treatment by psychiatrists and psychologists. It is to be hoped that psychiatric interest in rehabilitation will lead other members of the rehabilitation team to take on increasing responsibility for psychological components of treatment.

**REFERENCES**
1. Wenger, N., Hellerstein, H.K., Blackburn, H., Castranova, S.J. Circulation 65: 421-427, 1982.
2. Mayour, R.A., Foster, A., Williamson, B. J. Psychosom. Res. 22: 447-453, 1978.
3. Ruberman, W., Weinblatt, E., Goldberg, J.D., Chaudhary, B.S. New Eng. J. Med. 311: 552-559, 1984.
4. Taylor, C.B., Houstine-Miller, N., Ahn, D.K., et al. J. Psychosom Res. 30: 581-587.
5. Mayou, R.A. J. Psychosom. Res. 28: 17-25, 1984.
6. Mayou, R.A. Postgrad. Med. J. 49: 250-254, 1973.
7. Mayou, R.A. J. Psychosom. Res. 30: 255-271, 1986.
8. Mayou, R.A., Bryant, B.M. In Press, 1987.
9. Kannel, W.B. In: (eds) Wenger, N.K., Hellerstein, H.K. Rehabilitation of the Coronary Patient. Second edition. USA: John Wiley and Sons Inc. 1984.
10. Wenger, N., Hellerstein, H.K. Rehabilitation of the coronary patient. Second edition. USA: John Wiley and Sons Inc. New York. 1984.
11. Oldridge, N.B. J. Cardiopul. Rehab. 6: 153-156, 1986.
12. Gloag, D. Brit. Med. J. 290: 617-620, 1985.
13. Mitchell, J.R.A. Brit. Med. J. 285: 1140-1148, 1982.
14. De Busk, R., Blomqvist, G., Kouchoukos, N.T., et al. New Eng. Med. J. 314: 161-166, 1986.

15. Stern, M.J., Cleary, P.   Arch. Intern. Med.   142: 1093-1097, 1982.
16. Assal, J.P., Mühlhauser, I., Pernet, A., et al.   Diabetalogia. 28: 602-613.
17. Mathews, A., Ridgeway, V.   In: (eds) Steptoe, A., Matthews A. Health Care and Human Behavior. Academic Press. London. 1984.
18. Tuckett, D., Boulton, M., Olson, C., Williams, A.   Meetings between Experts. Tavistock Publications, London.  1985.
19. Wenger, N., Cleeman, J., Herd, A., McIntosh, H.  Am. J. Cardiol. 57: 1187-1189, 1986.
20. Johnston, D.W.  J. Psychosom. Res. 29: 447-456, 1985.
21. Kolman, P.B.R.  J. Cardiac Rehab. 3: 360-366, 1983.
22. Friedman, M., Thoresen, C.E., Gill, J.J., et al.  Am. Heart J. 112: 653-665, 1986.
23. Taylor, C.B., De Busk, R.F., Davidson, D.M., et al.  J. Chron. Dis. 34: 127-133, 1981.
24. Dennis, C.A., Miller, N.H., Schwartz, G., et al.  Circulation 74: supp 1, 9, 1986.

# 14

**MANAGEMENT OF RISK FACTORS**

Pekka Puska

Department of Epidemiology, The North Karelia Project, National Public Health Institute, Mannerheimintie 166, 00280 Helsinki, Finland

## GENERAL CONCEPTS

Extensive research during the last few decades has identified a few factors that predict atherosclerotic cardiovascular disease in a strong, consistent and independent way.

These causal factors are elevated serum LDL-cholesterol, smoking and elevated blood pressure and these factors are called the primary risk factors. In addition, physical inactivity, diabetes and certain psychosocial factors are commonly related to CVD. Prevention or correction of these factors form the basis for primary prevention of atherosclerotic disease (1).

Although primary prevention is the ideal alternative, secondary prevention is of great importance. Almost half of coronary deaths occur among people who already have obvious signs of the disease. Much research has been carried out to identify factors that predict death, recurrent attacks or other severe complications after the initial coronary attack.

During the period immediately after acute myocardial infarction, factors related to the size of the infarct are the chief determinants of mortality. After an initial period of high early mortality, the above mentioned primary risk factors seem to play a role. These primary risk factors probably predict recurrent attacks and deaths in longer term follow-up of survivors of myocardial infarction. Combining information on these factors with information on relevant signs and symptoms, it is possible to identify patients with excess risk (2).

Although relatively little hard evidence is available on the utility of correcting many of the risk factors following myocardial infarction, good management of them seems rational and without great hazard. Smokers should definitely be advised to quit, and comprehensive multifactorial management along with careful surveillance and management has been found to lower the rate of new coronary events (3). A Finnish study showed that after a secondary preventive intervention emphasizing health education, three years' cumulative coronary mortality was significantly smaller (18.6%) than in the randomized control group (29.4%) among myocardial infarction patients (4).

The current medical advice on risk factor control among survivors of myocardial infarction can be stated as follows:

1. Stop smoking as evidence shows a reduction in mortality in those who stop (5).
2. Control hypertension.
3. Reduce weight if obese as 2 & 3 will reduce myocardial work.

Supervised exercise and lipid control may be helpful in reducing the rate of new coronary events, but evidence of efficacy is still limited (6).

## THE BEHAVIORAL FRAMEWORK FOR RISK FACTOR MANAGEMENT

Once the medical knowledge to identify the needed risk factor management has been applied the task usually becomes a behavioral one. This is because the needed measures are mainly behavioral in terms of lifestyle changes or compliance to prescribed medical therapy.

Medical practice has long been based on the notion that after identification of the behavioral factors related to disease, mere informing the subjects (giving them knowledge) is sufficient to change behavior. Numerous studies and everyday practice show that this is seldom the case. Behavior has complex background and is embedded in the social and physical environment.

Inspite of the obvious problems there is little doubt that health behaviors can often be influenced among individuals and groups through active intervention. The degree of success depends on 1) the recipient, 2) the contents and intensity of the intervention, and 3) several situational factors. Amongst these factors, personal experience of the disease, possible sustained symptoms and threat of severe complications tend to favor necessary behavioral changes among MI patients. The problem lies in maintaining these changes over a long period of time.

For any major long-term changes it is important to realize that health behaviors form an essential part of the general lifestyle and are closely associated with the cultural background, technological development and socioeconomic situation of the community. Thus a comprehensive framework of strategies with appreciation of the community setting is needed.

There are several general models that may be applied to planning risk factor control activities aimed at changing health-related behaviors. The framework presented below has been used in the North Karelia project and is compatible with several aspects of these models (7,8). The framework of goals is as follows:

1. Information to educate people about the relationship between their behavior and disease (e.g. the health consequences of various aspects of the diet and the benefits of suggested changes).
2. Persuasion designed to convince people to take healthy action for changing their behaviors.
3. Training to increase skills of self-control, environmental management and social action for recommended behaviors.
4. Social support to help maintain the healthier habits.
5. Environmental change to create opportunities for healthy actions (to make the healthier choice the easier one).

Information

Cooperation with any advice depends greatly on the extent to which the people are informed about the purposes and importance of desired action. This may mean informing people about the relationship between certain behaviors and the disease and its complications and how the risks can be reversed through appropriate measures and by explaining the bases and principles of these measures. The design of effective information interventions can be facilitated by the application of practical principles derived from communication research and theory.

The messages must be simple and frequently repeated if they are to be comprehended and retained. The messages should be compatible with the local cultural norms and should be practical and clear. The role of interpersonal communication should be appreciated. Personal contacts and discussions are usually more effective than impersonal communication or written materials. Written materials should be well tested, have their behavioral objectives specified and fit the local culture. The impact of information dissemination is at its best, if new information concerning health and lifestyle has to be communicated to people. This is, however, seldom the case with the risk factors.

## Persuasion

Health-related behaviors are not usually changed simply by providing information. People often need to be persuaded to act on the information they have been given. A personal experience of myocardial infarction gives a firm basis for the persuasive action by doctors and other health personnel. There is a great deal of research and theory concerning the social psychology of persuasion. The "communication" approach focuses on process of communication. It emphasizes the power of the source of a persuasive message or how the message form or content influences cognitive processes in a human receiver. The "affective" approach to persuasion concentrates on emotional aspects. It emphasizes positive goals and positive emotional associations. The "behavioral" approach centers on achieving behavioral change with the assumption that attitudes and beliefs will follow. It is important to set achievable goals. Achievement of these will hopefully lead to positive experiences and increase in self-confidence.

## Training for Practical Skills

Persuasion is often sufficient to promote simple behavioral changes. But, when complex changes are recommended, as is the case for example with nutrition, it is not always easy to translate intention into action. Many subjects wish to change their eating habits but they lack adequate personal skills to do so. Because of such difficulties, interventions must go beyond education and persuasion to provide training, such as teaching people how to make complex challenging changes in their diets. Four basic steps appear necessary for optimal training: a) modelling or demonstration of new dietary patterns, b) guided and increasingly independent practice in those thoughts and actions, c) feedback concerning the appropriateness of responses and d) reinforcement in the form of support and encouragement that can be gradually withdrawn as the new habit or skill is well established.

## Social Support

No matter how effectively a subject has been taught, persuaded or trained to make healthy changes in their behavior, it is unlikely that the changes will be maintained unless they are reinforced by a supportive social environment. Sustained improvement of health behavior requires social support by the family and other influential groups of the subject. Thus risk factor management of MI patients should always involve the family in an appropriate way. Social support can also be arranged for therapeutic purposes by creation of groups for certain intervention purposes. Weight reduction is usually markedly facilitated by weight reduction groups where group pressures exercise strong social support to the group members. Such groups have also the advantage of using the "strength or weak ties", that is somewhat alien people have often greater influence in thoughts and behaviors than a very close person like a spouse.

## Environmental Modification

The environment has a determining influence on behavior through the opportunities and constraints that it provides. Thus a very important aspect of dietary counselling is to pay attention to the prevailing environemtnal options. Patients can be advised to pay attention to and sometimes to modify the environment relevant to risk factor control. In the long term the creation of consumer demand for new products or services can have powerful influence on environmental changes. In community-based programmes nutrition educators can and should approach directly representatives of agriculture, food industry, sales organizations and restaurants.

Finally, it should be pointed out that in principle, risk factor management of MI patients relates to the risk factor reductions needed in the population for primary prevention and health promotion.

Thus, organizing behavior risk factor management programs among patients should be ideally linked with related community actions. Risk factors among patients are closely and strongly linked with general lifestyle of that community. Thus to support desired long-term behavioral changes, ultimately the whole community should be involved and a social process promoting such changes should be achieved. It should be realized that patients are often strong opinion leaders on these matters in the community, as they tend frequently to talk about these issues and about what they think are important factors.

## WHICH RISK FACTOR REDUCTION STRATEGY TO CHOOSE?

At the same time as many agree with the above mentioned or related general theories, clinicians and program managers still have to make practical choices concerning the actual methods and strategies to be chosen for their particular needs in risk factor management. The question arises about the relative effectivenss of the different methods and strategies.

Many studies have assessed the effects of various intervention programs. Some have even compared the effectiveness of different approaches. Unfortunately, this helps little in the actual decision situation. The problem lies there that the effect is so much dependent, not only upon the method, but also upon the health worker and the target population, upon time and place etc. In addition to the effects one has to consider the feasibility of different strategies in the local situation. One has to consider the relationship between the costs involved and the effects desired. One has to consider the overall acceptability and broad aspects of possible consequences of the strategy chosen.

Thus it is obvious that no universally valid method can be recommended. However, some further general guidelines can be given.

Too often interventions are started without examining the behavioral background of the problem. As disease can be treated only after proper diagnosis, behavioral changes can be achieved only after identification of the determinants of desired changes. The following list gives some recommendations for diagnosis and subsequent action plan of behavior modification:

a.  describe the problem:  what behavior changes are needed?

b.  identify the history of the problem:  how long?  previous experiences?

c.  identify the present dynamics:  knowledge, beliefs, motivation, intentions

d.  aim at behavioral diagnosis:  where is the greatest problem?

e.  outline the action plan together:  step-by-step, achievable goals

f.  follow the progress and give positive feedback:  agreed follow-up days, record keeping, encouragement

It is obvious that any intervention program should combine different methods paying special attention to aspects of the feasibility and special features of the program and the patients. Below are listed several selected methods that commonly contribute to possible effects in risk factor modification programs:

a.  increased health knolwedge:  behaviors - health risks

b.  initial commitment:  promise, competition

c.  realistic action plan:  achievable gradual goals

d.  self monitoring:  record keeping

e.  encouragement and support:  follow-up and positive support by doctor and other health workers

f.  social support groups:  family, work-site group, other groups

g.  guided practical learning:  cooking, new recipes

h.  environment and stimulus control:  to minimize factors that support undesired behaviors

i.  relaxation and desensitization:  to help overcome withdrawal or other problems related to major behavioral change

j.  learning thoughts and self-reward:  positive thoughts, symbolic and material rewards

An important further consideration is the role of the different professionals. While the cardiologist and other medical doctors have clearly the highest authority and should thus initiate and strongly encourage the needed behavioral changes, other professionals can have a major role in the practical implementation of these changes. Nurses have often more time and the patients can more freely discuss the practical issues with them. Dietitians can teach the patients the practical ways to achieve recommended dietary changes, and psychologists can advise patients to achieve more demanding behavioral changes. Family members and other lay people can also be used in the health education of the patients.

It must be repeatedly pointed out that patients' habits are strongly influenced by the social and physical environments. Thus any behavior modification intervention not paying attention to this basic law is likely to have only a limited or no-long-term impact. In larger programmes the community-based approach has greatest potential for long-term and sustained change, as the experience from the North Karelia project in Finland has shown (8,9). In relation to myocardial infarction patients, several factors favor at least some success: a) the personal disease experience and threat of new attack, b) limited number of relatively high risk subjects, c) frequent visits to doctor and other health workers, and d) obvious concern of family members, etc. If this is combined by observing sound behavioral principles and personal dedication of professionals, major success in health education for risk factor management can be expected.

## REFERENCES

1. WHO, Technical Report Series 678. Geneva, 1982.
2. Kannel, W.B., Sorlie, P., McNamara, P.M. Am. J. Cardiol. 44: 53-59, 1979.
3. Vedin, A., Wilhelmsson, C., Tibblin, G., Wilhelmsen, L. Acta. Med. Scand. 200: 453-456, 1976.
4. Kallio, V., Hämäläinen, H., Hakkila, J., Luurila, O.J. Lancet ii: 1091-1094, 1979.
5. Salonen, J.T. Br. Heart J. 43: 463-469, 1980.
6. Kannel, W.B. In: Prevention of Coronary Heart Disease (Eds. Kaplan & Stamler), W.B. Saunders Company, Philadelphia, London, Toronto, Mexico City, Rio de Janeiro, Sydney, Tokyo p. 1-19, 1983.
7. McAlister, A., Puska, P., Salonen, J.T., et al. Am. J. Public Health 72(1): 43-50, 1982.
8. Pushka, P., Nissinen, A., Tuomilehto, J., et al. Ann. Rev. Public Health 6: 147-193, 1985.
9. Puska, P., Salonen, J.T., Nissinen, A., et al. Br. Med. J. 287: 1840-1844, 1983.

# 15

BENEFITS OF EXERCISE:   EFFECT ON MORTALITY AND PHYSIOLOGICAL FUNCTION

Michael L. Pollock

Center for Exercise, University of Florida, Gainesville, Florida, USA

## ABSTRACT

The effect of exercise on mortality from coronary heart disease (CHD) is equivocal.  Primary prevention studies have shown favorable results regarding persons who are active at work or during leisure time compared to sedentary persons.  However, non-randomization and sample selection problems make their validity questionable.  More recent evidence from Morris (1-3) on civil servants and Paffenbarger (4-7) on longshoremen and Harvard graduates provide stronger evidence for physical activity as an independent risk factor.  Of the nine randomized trials concerning cardiac rehabilitation after myocardial infarction (MI), seven showed inconclusive results (8-14), while two showed a favorable effect (15,16).  The two favorable studies had multiple interventions (low cholesterol diet and/or smoking cessation), and thus, could not provide conclusive evidence for an independent effect of exercise.  High dropout/cross over rates, small sample size, sample selection, and modest exercise protocols make data difficult to interpret.

Data concerning  the effect of exercise on risk factors are encouraging and suggest that exercise affects mortality from CHD. Exercise of the appropriate frequency, intensity and duration has had a favorable effect on cardiorespiratory function of healthy adults and cardiac patients.  While healthy adults show both central and peripheral adaptations to endurance training, cardiac patients improve mainly through peripheral adaptation.  More recent data from Ehsani (17,18) show that MI patients increased central function (rate pressure  product,  left  ventricular  ejection  fraction  and contractility) with high intensity training (@ 18 miles/wk at 85-90% of max). These patients showed less ST-segment depression and symptoms at a higher rate of pressure product. Although these data are provocative, the fact that high intensity exercise and training in patients who show significant ST-depression is associated with a greater incidence of cardiac arrest and mortality cannot be ignored. Future programs will need to better differentiate patients into high and low risk categories. This stratification should improve the patients capability of attaining their maximum potential physiological benefit without a greater risk of a cardiac event.

The purpose of this paper is to briefly review the effect of exercise or physical activity on mortality from coronary heart disease (CHD). Although emphasis will be placed on the secondary prevention trials, some recent work on primary prevention will be discussed. The question as to whether adaptive changes in both central and peripheral function occur as a result of exercise of the cardiac patients will also be reviewed.

## EXERCISE AND MORTALITY FROM CORONARY HEART DISEASE

### Primary Prevention

Most reports from epidemiological studies show favorable results concerning mortality from CHD when comparing populations of active individuals vs. their sedentary counterparts (19,20). However, these studies are non-randomized and tend to have methodological problems that limit the generalization of the results.

The issue of non-randomization is an important factor which leads to the question as to whether the more active and healthy individuals selected the more active jobs in the first place? This was certainly the case in the original study of Morris et al (1) who reported that conductors who moved vigorously around two tier London buses had a lower incidence of CHD than the sedentary drivers. Later, it was noted that the drivers uniform size was two inches larger around the waist than the conductors at job entry (2).

Other confounding factors that make the interpretation of most studies difficult is the lack of knowledge of other risk factors associated with CHD mortality, and of leisure-time activity habits.

Since most job classifications are rather sedentary, leisure-time activity may account for a larger proportion of the energy cost of daily activity.

More recently, the studies of longshoremen in San Francisco by Paffenbarger et al (4,5), of civil servants by Morris et al (2,3), and of Harvard graduates by Paffenbarger et al (5,6), have alleviated some of the pitfalls of previous studies. The study of longshoremen included a 22 year follow-up of 3,686 men (4). All subjects were screened for cigarette smoking, blood pressure, history of prior CHD, obesity, glucose intolerance and cholesterol. Death rates from fatal heart attacks were significantly lower for workers who had high energy cost jobs ( > 5.2 Kcal/min or > 8,500 Kcal/week) compared to workers with low energy cost jobs ( < 5.0 Kcal/min or < 8,500 Kcal/week). Thirty one percent of the man-years of work in the 22 year follow-up period was from workers in the high energy output group. The data also showed that workers with high energy cost jobs had less risk of sudden death from a heart attack and a reduced risk among workers with prior known heart disease. The effect was strongest among men less than 55 years of age but important in all age groups studied. The fact that the relationship between physical activity and a decrease in CHD death remained significant after other risk factors for CHD were statistically accounted for and that an inverse relationship between physical activity and CHD death was established makes this a landmark investigation.

Chave et al. (21) and Morris et al. (3) assessed the leisure-time activity habits of 17,944 male executive grade civil servants who were between 40 and 65 years of age. Executives who reported vigorous exercise over a two day sampling period (one week day and one weekend day) showed fewer heart attacks and deaths from CHD. This prospective study had an average subsequent follow-up of 8.5 years. Vigorous exercise was defined as "work liable to require peaks of energy expenditure of 7.5 Kcals per minute or more." Estimates of leisure-time in itself, without the vigorous component did not show a relationship with CHD. Although multivariate analysis was not used (3), the relationship between vigorous exercise, and fatal and non-fatal heart attacks and symptoms of CHD remained significant when family history, height-weight, cigarette smoking, hypertension, cholesterol, and diabetes mellitus were compared.

Paffenbarger et al. (5,6) investigated the leisure-time exercise habits and health status of 16,936 Harvard male graduates aged 35-74 years of age. Subjects entering college between 1916-1950 were assessed by initial physical examinations, self assessed mail questionnaires, and official death certificates. The follow-up period was from 6-10 years (1962 or 1966 to 1972) and 12-16 years (1962 or 1966 to 1978) for the two studies (5,6). Age specific rates for fatal and non-fatal cardiac events (angina pectoris, myocardial infarction (MI), and sudden death) were inversely related to increased physical activity of up to 2,000 Kcal/week (Figure 1).

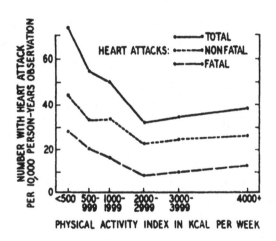

**FIGURE 1.** Age-adjusted first heart attacks; by physical activity index in 6-10 year follow-up of Harvard male alumni (5). Published with permission.

Men who expended less than 2,000 Kcal/week of extra effort during leisure-time were at a 64% higher risk of having an event resulting from CHD than men above that value. Approximately 33% of the alumni reported activity levels above the 2,000 Kcal/week. Vigorous sport/exercise enhanced the relationship between risk of first heart attack and physical activity. Thus, intensity of effort further increased the benefit derived from physical activity.

Athletes who were active earlier in life and who discontinued their exercise habits tended to be at a higher risk for CHD events than persons who remained sedentary their full life. Multivariate analyses for estimating death rates showed exercise to be an independent risk factor for CHD even when adjusted for age, cigarette smoking, early parental death from CHD, body weight gains, total body weight, and hypertension. In the 1986 publication, Paffenbarger et al. (7) showed that exercise alone accounted for up to two or more years of additional life.

In summary, Paffenbarger (7) concluded the following pertinent findings from the most recent studies:

"1. A reduced risk of developing CHD is related to both occupational and leisure-time aerobic practices of vigorous activity. A reduced CHD risk associated with an adequate level of current energy expenditure is lowered further if exercise pattern included sufficient vigorous activity or strenuous burst of energy output.

2. The relationship is dose dependent over a wide range; that is the greater energy expenditure . . . , the lower the incidence, case fatality, mortality, and recurrence.

3. The findings are consistent by age of subjects, by sex, and by clinical manifestation of disease (angina pectoris, myocardial infarction, sudden unexpected death, and fatal CHD death).

4. The findings persist over successive increments of time and in careful studies of several diverse populations cited here.

5. The findings for exercise influence are at least partially independent of other host and environmental characteristics associated with CHD risk (smoking, blood pressure level, weight-for-height status, prior existence of diabetes mellitus, family history of CHD, etc.)."

Secondary Prevention

There are nine randomized clinical trials that evaluate the efficacy of exercise or a combination of exercise and other lifestyle modifications, e.g. cigarette smoking cessation and diet modification, on mortality from CHD. Table 1 lists the nine studies including information on years of follow-up, sample size, percent mortality and statistical significance. In general, the follow-up period averaged 3.0-4.0 years and the sample size from 150-300 patients in the control and rehabilitation groups. Of the nine trials, only two showed positive results; Kallio et al. (15) had a significant reduction in mortality, and Vermuelen et al. (16) demonstrated a reduced mortality in combination with a lower progression of CHD in the rehabilitation group compared to the controls.

**TABLE 1.** Mortality results from randomized controlled trials of cardiac rehabilitation following myocardial infarction

| Trial (Year) | Follow-up (Year) | GROUPS Control n | Control Death | Rehabilitation n | Rehabilitation Death | P-Value ** |
|---|---|---|---|---|---|---|
| Kentala (1972) | 1.0 | 146 | 21.9 | 152 | 17.1 | NS |
| Wilhemsen (1975) | 4.0 | 157 | 22.3 | 158 | 17.7 | NS |
| Palatsi (1976) | 3.2(C)* 3.7(R)* | 200 | 14.0 | 180 | 10.00 | NS |
| Kallio (1979) | 3.0 | 187 | 29.9 | 188 | 21.8 | SIG |
| Shaw (1981) | 3.0 | 328 | 7.3 | 323 | 4.6 | NS |
| Vermueulen (1983) | 5.0 | 51 | 14.5 | 47 | 11.6 | SIG |
| Carson (1983) | 2.1 | 152 | 14.0 | 151 | 8.0 | NS |
| Roman (1983) | 3.6 | 100 | 24.0 | 93 | 14.0 | NS |
| Rechnitzer (1983) | 4.0 | 354 | 7.3 | 379 | 9.5 | NS |

* R, rehabilitation group; C, control group
** NS, non significant; SIG, significant mortality differences between control and rehabilitation groups

It is interesting to note that the two trials that showed significant reductions in mortality and progression of disease had multiple interventions, including smoking and diet interventions, along with an informal exercise program. Both programs reduced saturated fats and cholesterol in the diet and showed a significant reduction in total cholesterol for patients in their respective treatment groups. The incidence of smoking cessation was similar for both treatment and control groups in both studies. Neither trial demonstrated a difference in physical work capacity between control and intervention groups; thus, it appears that the dietary modifications are the most important intervention. The importance of the dietary modifications found in the above two trials is consistent with the results from the Lipid Research Clinic trial on primary prevention in the reduction of serum cholesterol (22).

Thus, the data from the nine trials listed in Table I indicates that exercise in itself has no effect on mortality in secondary prevention of CHD. However, when evaluating the methodological problems associated with these trials, this may not be the case. Small sample size, drop out/cross over rate, patient selection, and an ineffective exercise regimen are some of the major problems with these trials. For example, the National Exercise and Heart Disease Project (NEHDP) was not designed to determine if physical activity could significantly affect mortality from CHD in patients with previous MI (11,23). It was estimated that 4,200 patients with previous MI's were necessary to answer this question. Like all the trials but one (14) shown in Table 1, the NEHDP showed a trend in favor of exercise in decreasing mortality from CHD. Oberman mentioned in the NEHDP study that if this trend favoring the exercise group was maintained and if they would have had 1,500 patients in the study, the finding would have been significant.

As a result of the small sample in each of the studies, May et al. (24) pooled the data from six of the trials listed in Table 1 (8-11,14) and found a 19% reduction (p $<$ .05) in mortality from CHD in the intervention group. More recently, Kent and Pollock (25) pooled the data from all nine trials and found the following results:

Cardiovascular mortality in 1,675 control patients = 14.2%

Cardiovascular mortality in 1,671 intervention patients = 9.0%

Chi Square = 20.4, p $<$ .001

Nonfatal recurrent MI in 1,675 control patients = 10.5%

Nonfatal recurrent MI in 1,671 intervention patients = 10.5%

Chi Square = 0.49, not significant

The overall conclusion from the pooled data was that cardiac rehabilitation which emphasizes exercise significantly reduces mortality, but has no effect in reducing nonfatal events.

Although the pooled data of the nine trials concerning the effect of cardiac rehabilitation on mortality from CHD indicate a significant difference, statisticians sometimes question the validity of this technique. The techniques of testing, selection of patients, monitoring and supervision of patients, follow-up period, etc. vary somewhat among trials and, therefore, data may not be appropriate to pool. Thus, the pooled analysis must be interpreted with caution.

There is no question that the high dropout rates and cross over rates associated with these trials significantly affects their results. For example, in the Goteborg trial (9) a 65% dropout was found in the exercise intervention group and many of the controls began training (approximately 25%). It is interesting to note that the results from the two years data of Sanne, Elmfeldt, and Wilhemsen (26) showed a significant difference in mortality in favor of the treatment group compared to the control group, but not at four years (9). It is felt that the continued adherence/cross over problem after two years could have affected the outcome. A minimum of 50% dropout rate has been experienced in most of the clinical trials (27,28). It appears that the continued lack of adherence and small sample size had the greatest effect on the results of these trials.

Patient selection can be a problem and may also have affected the results from a couple of studies. For example, in the Ontario Exercise-Heart Collaborative Study, the fatal reinfarction rate was approximately 2% per year which is considered low for MI patients (29). May et al. (24) in their review of the effectiveness of various intervention trials with MI patients (antiarrhythmic, lipid lowering, beta blocker, and anti-coagulant-platelet active drugs, and physical exercise trials) found that it was difficult to reduce mortality below 2% per year. Thus, if you start off with a population of very low risk patients, it would be difficult to demonstrate an improved prognosis (reduction in mortality) using any intervention.

In summary, the effect of chronic exercise on the reduction of mortality in secondary prevention from CHD is non-conclusive.

Although eight of the nine trials discussed showed favorable trends, only two trials had significant differences. Methodological problems, eg. small sample size, high dropout/cross over rates, patient selection, short follow-up periods, and ineffective exercise regimens appear to have affected the results. When sample size was enhanced by pooling data from the various trials, exercise became significant as an intervention tool. The probability of designing and conducting a trial to adequately test the question of mortality is low to impossible. The high financial cost and difficulty of finding enough patients that are willing to be randomized, thus affecting adherence/cross over, and being able to control for other medical or non-medical lifestyle factors make future studies prohibitive. In the meantime, there is enough direct and indirect evidence showing that exercise in itself favorably affects various risk factors associated with CHD; e.g. increasing HDL cholesterol, reducing blood pressure, reducing or maintaining body composition, etc., to justify exercise as an integral part of rehabilitation programs (30-36). Since diet modification, cigarette smoking cessation, as well as certain medication regimens, etc., are known to favorably affect risk of developing CHD (16,22,30,34,37-40), a multiple intervention program is strongly recommended.

## EXERCISE AND ITS EFFECT ON PHYSIOLOGICAL FUNCTION

The effect of chronic endurance exercise is shown in Table 2 for both healthy adults and cardiac patients. Aerobic capacity and submaximal capacity improve in most patients (36,41), including those with low left ventricular function (42-44). While it is well established that healthy adults adapt to endurance training with both peripheral and central function mechanisms (36,41,45), many have suggested that cardiac patients improve mainly through peripheral mechanisms (36,44,46-48).

In contrast to the above findings with cardiac patients, Ehsani et al. (17,18) and Hagberg et al. (49) have shown both central and peripheral training effects when patients were trained at a high intensity.

In an attempt to clarify the contrasting views as to how cardiac

**TABLE 2.** The Effect of chronic physical activity on cardiovascular function/aerobic fitness in healthy adults and cardiac patients.

| Variables | Units | Changes in Endurance Training | |
| --- | --- | --- | --- |
| | | Healthy Adult | Cardiac Patients |
| **Maximal Values** | | | |
| Oxygen uptake | $ml \cdot kg^{-1} \cdot min^{-1}$ | Increase | Increase |
| Cardiac output | L/min | Increase | Unchanged ? |
| Heart rate | beats/min | Unchanged--decrease | Unchanged |
| Stroke volume | ml | Increase | Unchanged |
| Arteriovenous oxygen difference | ml/100 ml blood | Increase | Increase |
| Systolic blood pressure | mm Hg | Unchanged | Unchanged |
| Rate pressure product | beats/min x mm Hg x $10^3$ | Unchanged | Unchanged |
| Endurance | sec | Increase* | Increase* |
| **Submaximal Values**** | | | |
| Oxygen uptake | $ml \cdot kg^{-1} \cdot min^{-1}$ | Unchanged--decrease | Unchanged--decrease |
| Cardiac output | L/min | Unchanged | Unchanged |
| Heart rate | beats/min | Decrease | Decrease |
| Stroke volume | ml | Increase | Increase ? |
| Systolic blood pressure | mm Hg | Decrease | Decrease |
| Rate pressure product | beats/min x mm Hg x $10^3$ | Decrease | Decrease |
| **Resting Values** | | | |
| Oxygen uptake | $ml \cdot kg^{-1} \cdot min^{-1}$ | Unchanged | Unchanged |
| Heart rate | beats/min | Decrease | Decrease |
| Systolic blood pressure | mm Hg | Unchanged--decrease | Unchanged--decrease |
| Diastolic blood pressure | mm Hg | Unchanged--decrease | Unchanged--decrease |
| Rate pressure product | beats/min x mm Hg x $10^3$ | Decrease | Decrease |

\* The performance will improve, i.e., performance at a given distance will decrease, and performance time on a treadmill or cycle ergometer will increase.

\*\* Same absolute workload

patients adapt to endurance training, the investigations of Froelicher et al. (44) and Ehsani and Hagberg et al. (17,18,49) will be discussed. In order to determine whether endurance training had an effect on myocardial perfusion or function (i.e., a central effect), Froelicher et al. (44) randomized 146 male patients with stable CHD into exercise (n=72) and control (n=74) groups for a period of one year. The groups averaged 53 years of age. The exercise group trained mostly by walking, but arm plus leg ergometry and jogging was performed by some. The training was three times per week for approximately 45 minutes per session. The average intensity for the year was 60% $\pm$ 10% of maximum heart rate (HR) reserve as described by Karvonen et al. (50). The program would be considered of moderate intensity, and representative of many programs conducted in North America. The intensity was thought to be of sufficient a level to elicit a significant training effect.

The results of the program showed that the exercise group elicited the typical adaptations associated with such a program: reduced resting HR; reduced HR, systolic blood pressure (BP) and rate pressure product (RPP) at a standard submaximal work load; increased maximum oxygen uptake ($VO_2$ max 18%); and no change in maximum HR, systolic BP, and RPP. Less angina pectoris and ST-segment depression was found during the standard submaximal work test, however the RPP also was significantly lower as a result of training. At similar RPP values (pre vs. post training tests), there was no change in symptoms or ST-segment depression. In general, no improvement was found in physiological variables that could be related to improvement in central function, i.e. RPP at maximum which correlates with myocardial blood supply, stroke volume, cardiac output, left ventricular ejection fraction (both at rest and during exercise) and thallium perfusion. A small but significant improvement in stroke volume and cardiac output was found in the trained patients who did not have angina. Also, thallium perfusion improved slightly in the exercise group who had angina. The improvement in thallium perfusion with the angina group is in agreement with animal studies which suggest ischemia stimulates collateral flow; thus, exercise may act as a facilitator of this response.

Ehsani et al. (17,18) in a series of experiments dating from 1981 to the present have demonstrated consistent significant effects on central function in MI patients who participated in high intensity training. The subjects for these investigations included 10 to 25 in the exercise groups and 10 to 14 in control groups. Although subjects were not randomized, they were initially of similar age (@ 52 yr), physical characteristics, fitness level ($VO_2$ max), and medical status. The controls could not participate in the formal program generally because they lived too far from the exercise center. The training of their patients was of similar intensity (50-70% of $VO_2$ max), duration, and frequency as described by Froelicher et al. (44) for the first three months. The next nine months differed significantly through training of higher intensity (80-90% of $VO_2$ max), greater frequency (5 days per week), and increased duration (50-60 minutes, exclusive of warm-up and cool down periods). An example of the rigorousness of the training (18) showed the runners to average $18.1 \pm 1.6$ miles per week at a peak training intensity of $89.4 \pm 1.3\%$ of $VO_2$ max during the last 3 months of training. With this higher volume/intensity of training, $VO_2$ max increased 35-40%. Their results clearly showed a significant improvement in markers of central function: increased stroke volume and maximum RPP; and increased left ventricular ejection fraction from rest to exercise only after the training period. The systolic BP-end-systolic volume relationship was shifted upward and to the left, with an increase in maximal systolic BP and a smaller end-systolic volume, suggesting an improved contractile state after training. Also, markers of ischemia showed improvement after training, i.e. reduced ST-segment depression at maximal effort (higher RPP after training) and significantly less angina. No changes were found in the control group.

These new findings of Ehsani and Hagberg et al. (17,18,49) are provocative but must be interpreted with caution. It appears that higher intensity programs provide a greater potential benefit for the patient, i.e. increased aerobic capacity, which include adaptations of both central and peripheral factors, than the more traditional light to moderate intensity exercise regimens. But it is also known

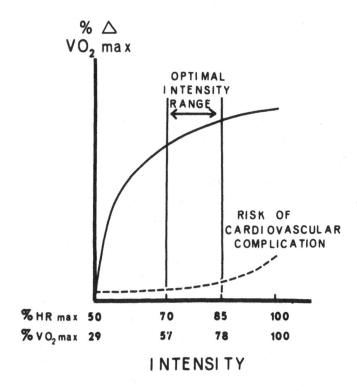

%Δ
VO₂ max

OPTIMAL
INTENSITY
RANGE

RISK OF
CARDIOVASCULAR
COMPLICATION

| %HR max | 50 | 70 | 85 | 100 |
| %VO₂ max | 29 | 57 | 78 | 100 |

INTENSITY

**FIGURE 2.** The relationship is shown between training intensity, percentage change in VO₂ max. and risk of cardiovascular complications (53). Published with permission.

that high intensity effort is associated with greater risk of precipitation of a major cardiac event (51-54). Hossack and Hartwig (52) found three significant factors that differentiated patients who required resuscitation from a major coronary event and those patients who did not during rehabilitation in the CAPRI program. Patients who had cardiac arrests had higher aerobic capacities, exercised more often above their recommended upper limit training HR, and had significant ST-segment depression of more than 1 mm of flat or downsloping ST-depression from the J point in response to exercise than the comparison group. Shephard et al. (55) reported that five of the first seven deaths in the Ontario Exercise-Heart Collaborative Study were in patients who showed deep ST-segment depression during exercise. Figure 2, from Hellerstein and Franklin (53) diagrammatically shows the relationship between exercise intensity (% $VO_2$ max), improvement in $VO_2$ max and risk of cardiovascular events. The figure shows a greater improvement in $VO_2$ max with increased intensity of training, and a dramatic increase in cardiovascular events when training exceeded 85% of $VO_2$ max. It must be emphasized that Ehsani (personal communication, 1985-1986) has had many patients training at a high intensity, 85-90% of $VO_2$ max, the past 5-6 years who had significant ST-segment depression during exercise and were without incident.

In summary, an interpretation of these results of improvement in physiological function with exercise training shows that most patients improve in functional capacity with exercise training. Low to moderate intensity programs show a greater benefit in $VO_2$ max and adaptation of both peripheral and central factors. Thus, it is important to treat patients individually, classifying them into high and low risk groups so that their training can be more specifically designed to allow them to be trained at a more appropriate intensity, but not at the cost of a greater risk of cardiovascular event. The current literature shows that high risk patients should be treated with greater caution and need more careful supervision. Classification of patients into low ($<$ 2% mortality per year) and high ($>$ than 5% mortality per year) risk groups has been defined by DeBusk et al. (29), Gillespie and Moss (56), and the American College of Sports Medicine (57) and can be used as a guide for patient classification. Certainly, exercising patients who show significant ST-segment depression, malignant types of arrhythmias (especially with patients who have left ventricular dysfunction, $<$ 35% ejection fractions), low functional capacities ($<$ 5 METs), poor systolic BP ($<$ 140 mm Hg) and HR response to exercise ($<$ 120 beats per minute without beta blocking drugs), as well as indications of medical instability should proceed more conservatively and with greater caution (29,58,59).

## REFERENCES

1. Morris, J.N., Heady, J.A., Raffle, P.A.B., et al. Lancet ii: 1053-1057, 1111-1120, 1953.

2. Morris, J.N., Heady, J.A., Raffle, P.A.B. Lancet ii: 569-570, 1956.
3. Morris, J.N., Pollard, R., Everitt, M.G., Chave, S.P.W. Lancet December: 1207-1210, 1980.
4. Paffenbarger, Jr., R.S., Hale, W.E., Brand, R.J., Hyde, R.T. Am. J. Epidemiol. 105: 200-213, 1977.
5. Paffenbarger, Jr., R.S., Wing, A.L., Hyde, R.T. Am. J. Epidemiol. 108: 161-175, 1978.
6. Paffenbarger, Jr., R.S., Hyde, R.T., Wing, A.L., Hsieh, C. N. Engl. J. Med. 314: 605-613, 1986.
7. Paffenbarger, Jr., R.S. Exercise in the Primary Prevention of Coronary Heart Disease. In: M.L. Pollock and D.H. Schmidt (Eds.), Heart Disease and Rehabilitation, 2nd Edition, New York: John Wiley, p. 349-368, 1986.
8. Kentala, E. Ann. Clin. Res. 4 (Suppl 9): 1-84, 1972.
9. Wilhemsen, L., Sanne, H., Elmfeldt, D., et al. Preventive Medicine 4: 491-508, 1975.
10. Palatsi, I. Acta Medica Scandinavica 559 (Suppl): 1-84, 1976.
11. Shaw, L.W. Am. J. Cardiol. 48: 39-46, 1981.
12. Carson, P., Phillips, R., Lloyd, M., et al. J. Royal College of Physicians of London 16: 147-151, 1982.
13. Roman, O., Gutierrez, M., Luksic, I., et al. Cardiology 70: 223-231, 1983.
14. Rechnitzer, P.A., Cunningham, D.A., Andrew, G.M., et al. Am. J. Cardiol. 51: 65-69, 1982.
15. Kallio, V., Hamalainen, H., Hakkila, J., Luurila, O.J. Lancet November: 1091-1094, 1979.
16. Vermeulen, A., Lie, K.I., Durrer, D. Am. Heart J. 105: 798-801, 1983.
17. Ehsani, A.A., Heath, G.W., Hagberg, J.M., et al. Circulation 64: 1116-1124, 1981.
18. Ehsani, A.A., Biello, D.R., Shultz, J., et al. Circulation 74: 350-358, 1986.
19. Fox, S.M., Skinner, J.S. Am. J. Cardiol. 14: 731-746, 1964.
20. Froelicher, V.F., Oberman, A. Progress in Cardiov. Dis. 15: 41-55, 1972.
21. Chave, S.P.W., Morris, J.N., Moss, S., Semmence, A.M. J. Epidemiol. & Community Health 32: 239-243, 1978.
22. Lipid Research Clinic Program. JAMA 251: 351-364, 1984.
23. Oberman, A., Naughton, J. The National Exercise and Heart Disease Project. In: M.L. Pollock and D.H. Schmidt (Eds.), Heart Disease and Rehabilitation (2nd Edition), New York: John Wiley, p. 369-385, 1986.
24. May, G.S., Eberlein, K.A., Furberg, C.D., et al. Prog. Cardiov. Dis. 24: 331-352, 1982.
25. Kent, L.K., Pollock, M.L. (Chairman) (In Press) J. Cardiopulmonary Rehabilitation.
26. Sanne, H., Elmfeldt, D., Wilhelmsen, L. Preventive Effect of Physical Training After a Myocardial Infarction. In: G. Tibblin, A. Keys, and L. Werko (Eds.), Preventive Cardiology, John Wiley: New York, p.154-160, 1972.
27. Oldridge, N.B. Adherence to Adult Exercise Fitness Programs. In: J.D. Matarazzo, S.M. Weiss, J.A. Herd, et al. (Eds.), Behavior Health: A Handbook of Health Enhancement and Disease

Prevention, New York: John Wiley, p. 467-487, 1984.

28. Oldridge, N.B. Preventive Medicine 11: 56-70, 1982.

29. DeBusk, R.F., Blomqvist, C.G., Kouchoukos, N.T., et al. N. Engl. J. Med. 314: 161-166, 1986.

30. Wood, P.D., Haskell, W.L., Blair, S.N., et al. Metabolism 32: 31-39, 1983.

31. Hubert, H.B., Feinleib, M., McNamera, P.M., Castelli, W.P. Circulation 67: 968-977, 1983.

32. Seals, D.R., Hagberg, J.M. Medicine and Science in Sports and Exercise 16: 207-214, 1984.

33. American College of Sports Medicine. Medicine and Science in Sports and Exercise 15: ix-xiii, 1983.

34. Leon, A.S., Conrad, J., Hunninghake, D.B., Serfass, R. Am. J. Clin. Nutrition 33: 1776-1787, 1979.

35. Pollock, M.L., Schmidt, D.H., editors. Heart Disease and Rehabilitation, 2nd Edition, New York: John Wiley, 1986.

36. Astrand, P.O., Rodahl, K.. Textbook of Work Physiology (3rd Edition), New York: McGraw-Hill, 1986.

37. Arntzenius, A.C., Kromhout, D., Barth, J.D., et al. N. Engl. J. Med. 312: 805-811, 1985.

38. Kushi, L.H., Lew, R.A., Stare, F.J., et al. N. Engl. J. Med. 312: 811-818, 1985.

39. Kornitzer, M., Dramaix, M., Thilly, C., et al. Lancet May: 1066-1070, 1983.

40. Hjermann, I., Holme, I., Velve Byre, K., Leren, P. Lancet December: 1303-1310, 1981.

41. Pollock, M.L., Wilmore, J.H., Fox, S.M. Exercise in Health and Disease: Evaluation and Prescription for Prevention and Rehabilitation, Philadelphia: W.B. Saunders, 1984.

42. Lee, A.P., Ice, R., Blessey, R., Sanmarco, M.E.. Circulation 60: 1519-1526, 1979.

43. Conn, E.H., Williams, R.S., Wallace, A.G. Am. J. Cardiol. 49: 296-300, 1982.

44. Froelicher, V., Jensen, D., Genter, F., et al. JAMA 252: 1291-1297, 1984.

45. Haskell, W.L. Mechanisms by Which Physical Activity May Enhance the Clinical Status of Cardiac Patients. In: M.L. Pollock and D.H. Schmidt (Eds.), Heart Disease and Rehabilitation (2nd Edition), New York: John Wiley, p.303-324, 1986.

46. Clausen, J.P., Trapp-Jensen, J. Circulation 42: 611-624, 1970.

47. Clausen, J.P. Prog. Cardiovasc. Dis. 18: 459-495, 1976.

48. Foster, C., Pollock, M.L., Anholm, J.D., et al. Circulation 69: 748-755, 1984.

49. Hagberg, J.M., Ehsani, A.A., Holloszy, J.P. Circulation 67: 1194-1199, 1983.

50. Karvonen, M., Kentala, K., Musta, O. Ann. Med. Experimental Biology 35: 307-315, 1957.

51. Haskell, W.L. Circulation 57: 920-925, 1978.

52. Hossack, K.F., Hartwig, R., J. Cardiac Rehab. 2: 402-408, 1982.

53. Hellerstein, H.K., Franklin, B.A. Exercise Testing and Prescription. In: N.K. Wenger and H.K. Hellerstein (Eds.), Rehabilitation of the Coronary Patient (2nd Edition), New York: John Wiley, p. 197-284, 1984.

54. Shephard, R.J.. In: M.L. Pollock and D.H. Schmidt (Eds.), Heart Disease and Rehabilitation (2nd Edition), New York: John Wiley, p. 713-740, 1986.
55. Shephard, R.J., Kavanagh, T., Kennedy, J., Qureshi, S. British Journal of Sports Medicine 15: 6-16, 1981.
56. Gillespie, J.A., Moss, A.J. J. Am. Coll. Cardiol. 8: 50-51, 1986.
57. American College of Sports Medicine. Guidelines for Exercise Testing and Exercise Prescription (3rd Edition), Philadelphia: W.B. Saunders, 1986.
58. McNeer, J.F., Margolis, J.E., Lee, K.L., et al. Circulation 57: 64-70, 1978.
59. Froelicher, V.F., Perdue, S.T., Atwood, J.E., et al. Current Problems in Cardiology 11: 370-444, 1986.

# IV. FUTURE TRENDS

# 16

## CALCIUM CHANNEL BLOCKERS AND ISCHEMIA:  A REVIEW

Winifred G. Nayler, Wayne J. Sturrock and Sianna Panagiotopoulos

Department of Medicine, University of Melbourne, Austin Hospital, Heidelberg 3084, Victoria, Australia

### INTRODUCTION

This paper is primarily concerned with the use of calcium channel blockers for the long-term management of patients with ischemic heart disease.  The topic is timely, because whereas the recent clinical trials with beta adrenoceptor antagonists (1) and platelet inhibitors (2) have shown them to be effective under these conditions, comparable clinical trials with calcium channel blockers have, with one recent exception (3), yielded disappointing results (4-7).  The exception is the recently completed trial in which diltiazem was used (3).  At the outset it is important to note the essential differences between the diltiazem trial and the other calcium channel blocker trials, which involved either verapamil or nifedipine.  Firstly, the diltiazem study relates to a particular subset of patients - those with non-Q wave or non-transmural infarcts.  Secondly, treatment was not initiated until 24-72 hours after the onset of severe chest pain.  Thirdly, the trial lasted for only fourteen days, and used re-infarction as its end-point.  The most remarkable finding of this study was that whilst mortality was unchanged, the rate of re-infarction was reduced ($p < 0.03$).  Even though this trial involved a relatively small population of selected patients (3) and the period of follow up was limited, the results are important in that they show that in this particular subset of patients who are a high risk group for recurrent infarction (8-10), prophylactic therapy with this particular calcium channel blocker can slow, or prevent, the progression of damage caused by inadequate perfusion.  The results of this trial, therefore, substantiate the idea that calcium channel blockers (11-14) can protect the potentially jeopardized myocardium, provided that the appropriate therapy is initiated at the appropriate time, at the appropriate dose level, and to the appropriate patients.

The first of the calcium channel blocker/myocardial infarction trials to be completed was that carried out by Fischer-Hansen and his colleagues in Denmark (4,15). They started verapamil therapy within four hours of the onset of severe chest pain (Table 1) and continued treatment for up to 180 days. The trial was a relatively large study, involving 717 patients in the verapamil group and 719 in the placebo group.

**TABLE 1.** Clinical trials with calcium antagonists in myocardial infarction

| Calcium Antagonists | Patient Numbers | Time to Treat | Index of Response | Ref. |
|---|---|---|---|---|
| Diltiazem (D) | 289-D 282-P | 24 - 72 hrs | Re-infarction | (3) |
| Verapamil (V) | 717-V 719-P | 4 hrs | Mortality Re-infarction | (4,15) |
| | 25-V 25-P | 8 hrs | CK release | (17) |
| | 29-V 25-P | 7 ± 5 hrs | CK release | (5) |
| Nifedipine (N) | 115-N 112-P | 5.5 ± 2.9 hrs | CK release | (6) |
| | 89-N 82-P | 4.6 ± 0.1 hrs | CK release mortality | (6) |
| | 64-N 68-P | 8.0 ± 2.5 hrs | Mortality re-infarction | (7) |
| | 592-N 562-P | Admission to CCU | Mortlaity | (18) |

P = refers to placebo
Time to treat refers to the time interval between the onset of severe chest pain and the initiation of therapy.

On the basis of data obtained over 180 days of treatment verapamil failed to reduce the incidence of mortality (Table 1). On first inspection this is a discouraging result, but if the trial data is analysed in greater depth, then an interesting pattern emerges. In the first week of treatment the death rate was higher in the verapamil (6.4%) than in the placebo (5.6%) group. Death was due, usually, to cardiac failure, cardiogenic shock and arrhythmias. However, if the data that relates only to the 22-180 days to treatment is considered then mortality ($p < 0.03$) and the rate of re-infarction ($p < 0.05$) were both reduced (15). This trial seems to show, therefore, that for those patients who survive their first infarct and who are maintained on verapamil therapy, the risk of re-infarction is reduced. This is the same conclusion as was reached in the diltiazem study - where calcium channel blocker treatment was withheld for several days (3).

The data obtained from trials in which nifedipine has been used is complex and again quite difficult to analyse, sometimes because of an unusual patient selection, sometimes because of a significant increase in death rate (2.5% for placebo, 7.5% for nifedipine) in the early days of treatment, and sometimes because of the use of doses which were inappropriately low. There is, however, one particular nifedipine trial which warrants further attention, and that is the prospective double-blind randomized trial of Gerstenblith et al. (16). This trial was based on the assumption that persistent angina often progresses to infarction in patients who are placed on the traditional regime of beta-blockade and long acting nitrates. Gerstenblith's trial (16) extended over a period of four months, during which time it became apparent that the administration of nifedipine conferred benefit in that it reduced the incidence of death, myocardial infarction, or need for bypass surgery ($p < 0.03$) in a group of patients with unstable angina. This trial, therefore, in common with the other trials in which either verapamil (15) or diltiazem (3) was used, shows that the calcium channel blockers can reduce ischemic injury - or delay that injury, provided that the drugs are used as prophylactic agents.

**TABLE 2.** Laboratory Studies Showing Protection by Calcium Channel Blockers

| Species | Ischemia | Duration | Drug | Administration | Criteria | Follow up | Ref. |
|---|---|---|---|---|---|---|---|
| Dog | Regional | 40 min | V | Pre-occlusion | Infarct size | 4 days | 20 |
| | Regional | 1-2 min | N | Pre-occlusion | ECG; Mito. function | 105 days | 31 |
| | Regional | 1 hr | V | Pre-occlusion | Mito. and Mech-function | No reper. | 32 |
| | Regional | 15 min | V | Pre-occlusion | ATP | 24 hr | 33 |
| | Regional | 5-10 min | D | Pre-occlusion | Mito. function | No reper. | 34 |
| | Regional | 60 min | D | Pre-occlusion | Mito. function | 10 min | 12 |
| | Regional | 60 min | V | 30 min post occlusion | CK release | 24 hr | 21 |
| | Regional | 20-80 min | V/N | 20 min post occlusion | Segmental wall motion | 1 hr | 22 |
| Rat | Global | 27 min | V | Pre-occlusion | Mech-function; ATP/ADP | 30 min | 13 |
| | Global | 15 min | N | Pre-occlusion | ATP, Mech-function | 40 min | 35 |
| Swine | Regional | 75 min | D | Pre-occlusion | Infarct size; ATP | 4 hr | 36 |
| Rabbit | Global | 60 min | V | Pre-occlusion | Reduced $Ca^{2+}$ | 30 min | 37 |
| | Global | 60 min | N | Pre-occlusion | Reduced $Ca^{2+}$; ATP | 30 min | 23 |
| | Low flow ischemia | 60 min | V | Pre-occlusion | Mech-function; $Ca^{2+}$ gain; ATP | 60 min | 11,30 |

V = verapamil; N = nifedipine; D = diltiazem
Mito. function refers to mitochondrial respiratory activity
ATP refers to preservation of cardiac adenosine triphosphate (ATP)
CK release refers to plasma creatine kinase
Mech. function refers to contractility
$Ca^{2+}$ gain refers to increase in cardiac $Ca^{2+}$

LABORATORY STUDIES:  WHAT HAVE THEY SHOWN?

Irrespective of which particular calcium channel blocker has been used (Table 2), and irrespective of how the presence or absence of a protective effect has been quantitated (in terms of creatine kinase release, ST segment elevation, $Ca^{2+}$ gain, preservation of adenine precursors, maintenance of mitochondrial function, recovery

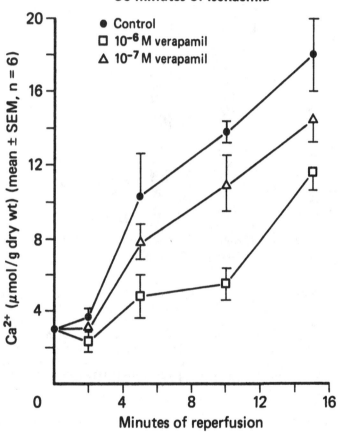

**Verapamil added on reperfusion after 30 minutes of ischaemia**

FIGURE 1.    Effect of adding verapamil ($10^{-6}$M and $10^{-7}$M) on reperfusion-induced $Ca^{2+}$ gain in isolated Langendorff perfused rat hearts reperfused after 30 minutes of ischemia at 37 degrees centigrade.    The perfusion buffer was Krebs-Henseleit solution. Verapamil was added only upon reperfusion, after the 30 minutes of global ischemia.  Each point is mean ± SEM of six separate studies.

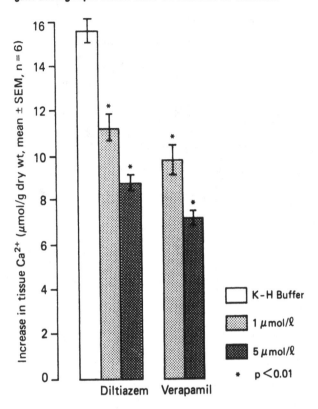

**FIGURE 2.** Effect of pretreatment with diltiazem and verapamil on reperfusion-induced $Ca^{2+}$ gain. The drugs were added 15 minutes before making the isolated rat hearts ischemic. Ischemia was produced by totally occluding coronary flow, but maintaining left ventricular wall temperature at 37 degrees centigrade. Tests of significance (analysis of variance) relates to the effectivness of diltiazem and verapamil in reducing reperfusion-induced $Ca^{2+}$ gain.

of contractility, measurement of infarct size, or maintenance of electrical stability) experimental studies in which these drugs have been introduced only after the coronary occlusive event, have failed to provide unequivocal evidence of protection. For example, excessive $Ca^{2+}$ gain is not avoided under these conditions (Fig. 1). This failure to protect when added after the occlusive event could have been anticipated, because the $Ca^{2+}$ channel blockers cannot reverse the ischemic-reperfusion-induced damage. They may however, prevent any damage which occurs early in the ischemic episode from progressing to an irreversible state.

Contrasting with the failure of these drugs to provide protection when added after the ischemic injury has progressed to the irreversible state, and the tissue is therefore doomed to die, is the data which shows evidence of protection, provided that the drugs are added prior to the ischemic episode. Verapamil (18-20), nifedipine (11,21-23) and diltiazem (12) have all been shown to be effective under such conditions. Fig. 2, for example, shows that when used in this way, as prophylactic agents, these drugs can protect in the sense of attenuating post-ischemic $Ca^{2+}$ overload.

If the slow channel blockers are to be used to provide effective prophylactic therapy for the long-term management of patients with ischemic heart disease, then it is important that any consequence of their long-term usage is recognized, that the pharmacodynamic profile of the compound ensures that sufficient drug is available for receptor binding on a twenty-four hour basis, and that the drug in question does not disrupt the metabolic dispersion of any other drugs.

Long-acting slow channel blockers are now available. They include the dihydropyridine derivative amlodipine, and the verapamil derivative, anipamil.

## SLOW CHANNEL BLOCKERS AND THE ISCHEMIC MYOCARDIUM

Ischemia has a profound effect on the myocardium. Peak developed tension rapidly declines, relaxation is impaired, the energy-rich phosphates are rapidly depleted, the glycolytic pathways are activated, ionic homeostasis is lost, tissue catecholamines are released, and the tissue becomes acidotic (24). If these ischemic conditions persist for more than a few minutes the subsequent re-introduction of perfusion precipitates an excessive and uncontrolled gain in $Ca^{2+}$ (Fig. 1 and 2), signalling cell death and tissue necrosis.

There are many reasons why an uncontrolled $Ca^{2+}$ gain signals cell death. Firstly, a raised cytosolic $Ca^{2+}$, even in the absence of adenosine triphosphate, will cause a sustained increase in end-diastolic resting tension, thereby indirectly impairing left ventricular filling, and further reducing flow through any vessels which are still patent. Other consequences of an uncontrolled $Ca^{2+}$ gain include the activation of the various ATPases, proteases and phospholipases - resulting in further ATP wastage, together with membrane disruption. Arachidonic acid production will also be stimulated, resulting in an even greater reduction in coronary flow. In addition much of the $Ca^{2+}$ that accumulates with the myocytes will be taken up by the mitochondria. Under such conditions the mitochondria will no longer be able to generate energy-rich phosphates, even through an unlimited supply of $O_2$ and substrates have been restored (11).

The data listed in Figs. 1 and 2 show quite clearly that the slow channel blockers can attenuate reperfusion-induced $Ca^{2+}$ overload, provided that the drugs are present prior to the ischemic episode. Recent investigations in our own laboratories indicate, however, that this ability to attenuate $Ca^{2+}$ overload may be only one facet of the mode of action of these drugs. Thus six weeks' therapy with orally-administered 50 mg/kg/day verapamil causes a highly significant reduction ($p < 0.001$) in the norepinephrine content of heart muscle (Table 3).

**TABLE 3.** Effect of prolonged therapy with verapamil on ventricular norepinephrine in spontaneously hypertensive (SHR), Wistar Kyoto (WKY) and Sprague Dawley (SD) rats.

| Species | Norepinephrine (mcg/g dry wt) | |
|---------|-------------------------------|-------------------------------|
|         | Placebo treated | Verapamil treated |
| SHR | $2.47 \pm 0.18$ | $0.86 \pm 0.06$ |
| WKY | $5.01 \pm 0.31$ | $0.93 \pm 0.10$ |
| SD | $3.85 \pm 0.30$ | $0.87 \pm 0.06$ |

Each result is mean + SEM of six separate determinations.
Verapamil (50 mg/kg/day) was given orally and provided a plasma level of 80-100 ng/ml.

Previously we (25) and others (26) have shown that ischemia promotes a release of endogenous norepinephrine from the myocardium (Fig. 3). Naturally, in the case of calcium channel blockers such as verapamil, if prolonged therapy has already depleted the endogenous norepinephrine reserves, then ischemia could no longer be expected to promote a large release of norepinephrine.

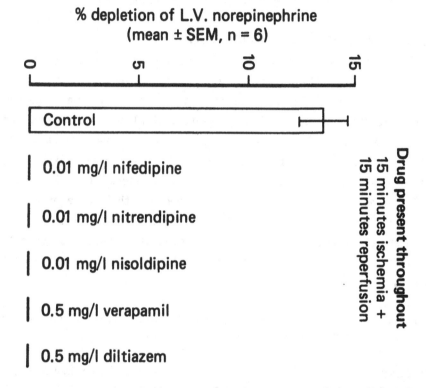

FIGURE 3. Effect of slow channel blockers on the release of norepinephrine caused by ischemia. Ischemia was for 15 minutes, at 37 degrees centigrade. Each bar is mean $\pm$ SEM of six separate experiments.

## CALCIUM CHANNEL BLOCKADE AND THE ATTENUATION OF EXCESSIVE $Ca^{2+}$ GAIN UPON REPERFUSION

If prophylactic therapy with $Ca^{2+}$ channel blockers attenuates reperfusion-induced $Ca^{2+}$ overload, and if such an effect is important in preserving tissue structure and function, then it is logical to question how the $Ca^{2+}$ channel blockers achieve such an effect. Probably it is an indirect consequence of their energy-sparing activity (11), together with their ability to slow the loss of adenosine precursors. It would be naive to suggest that the excessive entry of $Ca^{2+}$ that occurs upon reperfusion only involves entry through the slow channels, and it would be equally naive to assume that the $Ca^{2+}$ channel blockers directly block the major route of entry. If this was the case then these drugs would be effective when added only upon reperfusion, and they are not (Fig. 1).

## SLOW CHANNEL BLOCKERS AND ATHEROSCLEROSIS

The beneficial effect of slow channel-blocker therapy is not limited to their effect on $Ca^{2+}$ homeostasis, energy preservation (11) and norepinephrine storage. In addition, their long term usage can attenuate atherosclerotic plaque formation (Table 4) and even hasten its regression (27). This ability of slow channel blockers to attenuate atherosclerosis is shared by the phenylalkylamine, dihydrophyridine and benzothiazipeine - derivatives alike (28), but $Ca^{2+}$ channel blockade may be only one aspect of their mode of action in this respect. Thus at least one of these drugs hastens cholesterol catabolism (29). Some of them slow smooth muscle cell proliferation, a fundamental component of the atherosclerotic process.

**TABLE 4.** % Change in sudanophilic lesions after eight weeks treatment with Verapamil or Nifedipine.

| Treatment | % Change in Lesions |
|---|---|
| Verapamil (8 mg/kg/day, orally) | 65% decrease |
| Nifedipine (1 mg/kg/day, orally) | 38% decrease |
| Alpha methyl-dopa (8 mg/kg/day, orally) | 39% decrease |

Footnote: The rabbits (New Zealand White cross) were maintained on a hypercholesterolaemic diet for eight weeks, with and without drug therapy. Lesions were detected in the abdominal aorta, using Sudan IV staining. Rabbits which were not drug-treated but which were on the hypercholesterolaemic diet had 73% of their aorta covered with plaques. Note that the vasodilator drug alpha methyl-dopa did not reduce the number of Sudan IV positive lesions.

The calcium channel blockers are potent coronary vasodilators, a property which is of particular advantage under conditions in which the inadequate coronary blood flow is due to the presence of atherosclerotic plaques. The distribution of these plaques is such that they are seldom concentric. Under these conditions, as opposed to coronary underperfusion that is caused by a fixed stenosis, the coronary vasodilator effect of the calcium channel blockers will be of use, since dilation of the normal regions adjacent to the atherosclerotic plaque in the vascular wall will probably improve flow to the affected region.

## CONCLUSION

In conclusion, the successful use of the slow channel blockers in the management of ischemic heart disease necessitates prophylactic therapy. The proposed long-term usage of these drugs requires a careful appraisal of their long-term, as opposed to their acute effects. They are complex drugs with a remarkable degree of chemical heterogeneity, and whilst their predominant property is that of attenuating slow channel function, these drugs exhibit other properties which are difficult to account for in terms of slow channel blockade.

There appears to be no simple explanation for the ability of these drugs to attenuate ischemia - reperfusion induced damage. Their mode of action is probably multifactorial, and involves a direct effect on the myocytes and the vasculature.

Whereas these drugs cannot reverse the damage caused by prolonged ischemia, their prophylactic use can, under certain circumstances, slow the progression and reduce the intensity of that damage.

## ACKNOWLEDGEMENT

These investigations were supported by grants from the National Health and Medical Research Council of Australia, and the National Heart Foundation of Australia.

## REFERENCES
1. Yusuf, S., Peto, R., Lewis, J., et al. Cardiovasc. Dis. 27: 335-371, 1985.

2. Klimt, C.R., Knatterud, G.L., Stamler, J., Meier, P. J. Am. Coll. Cardiol. 7: 251-269, 1986.
3. Gibson, R.S., Boden, W.E., Theroux, P., et al. N. Engl. J. Med. 315: 423-429, 1986.
4. Danish Multicenter Study Group on Verapamil in Myocardial Infarction. Am. J. cardiol. 54: 24E-28E, 1984.
5. Crea, F., Deanfield, J., Crean, P., et al. Am. J. Cardiol. 55: 900-904, 1985.
6. Sirnes, P.A., Overskeid, K., Pedersen, T.R., et al. Circulation 70: 638-644, 1984.
7. Muller, J.E., Morrison, J., Stone, P.H., et al. Circulation 69: 740-747, 1984.
8. Marmor, A., Geltman, E.M., Schechtman, K., et al. Circulation 66: 415-421, 1982.
9. Geltman, E.M., Ehsani, A.A., Campbell, M.K., et al. Circulation 60: 805-814, 1979.
10. Gibson, R.S., Beller, G.A., Gheorghiade, M., et al. Circulation 73: 1186-1198, 1986.
11. Nayler, W.G., Ferrari, R., Williams, A. Am. J. Cardiol. 46: 242-248, 1980.
12. Weishaar, R.E., Bing, R.J. J. Mol. Cell. Cardiol. 12: 993-1009, 1980.
13. Watts, J.A., Maiorano, L.F., Maiorano, P.C. J. Mol. Cell. Cardiol. 17: 797-804, 1985.
14. Ferrari, R., Albertini, A., Curello, S. et al. J. Mol. Cell, Cardiol. 18: 487-498, 1986.
15. The Danish Study Group on Verapamil in Myocardial Infarction. Br. J. Clin. Pharmacol. 21: 197S-204S, 1986.
16. Gerstenblith, G., Ouyang, P., Achuff, S.C., et al. N. Engl. J. Med. 306: 885-889, 1982.
17. Bussman, W.D., Seher, W., Gruengras, M. Am. J. Cardiol. 54: 1224-1230, 1984.
18. Wilcox, R.G., Hampton, J.R., Banks, D.C., et al. Circulation 55: 581-587, 1977.
19. Reimer, K.A., Lowe, J.E., Jennings, R.B. Circulation 55: 581-587, 1977.
20. Reimer, K.A., Jennings, R.B. Lab Invest. 51: 655-666, 1984.
21. Henry, P.D., Shuchleib, R., Clark, R.E., Perez, J.E. Am. J. Cardiol. 44: 817-824, 1979.
22. Perez, J.E., Sobel, B.E., Henry, P.D. Am. J. Physiol. 239: H658-H663, 1980.
23. Nayler, W.G. J. Thorac. Cardiovasc. Surg. 84: 897-905, 1982.
24. Nayler, W.G., Elz, J.S. Circulation 74: 215-221, 1986.
25. Nayler, W.G., Sturrock, W.J. J. Cardiovasc. Pharmacol. 7: 581-587, 1985.
26. Holmgren, S., Abrahamsson, T., Almgren, O., Eriksson, B.M. Cardiovasc. Res. 15: 680-689, 1981.
27. Sievers, R., Rashid, T., Garrett, J., et al. J. Am. Coll. Cardiol. 7: 58A, 1986.
28. Henry, P.D. Circulation 72: 456-459, 1985.
29. Etingin, O.R., Hajjar, D.P. J. Clin. Invest. 75: 1554-1558, 1985.
30. Bersohn, M.M., Skine, K.I. J. Mol. Cell. Cardiol. 15: 659-671, 1983.

31. Fujibay, Y., Yamazaki, S., Chang, B., et al. J. Am. Coll. Cardiol. 6: 1289-1298, 1985.
32. Yoon, S.B., McMillin-Wood, J.B., Michael, L.H., et al. Circ. Res. 56: 704-708, 1985.
33. Lange, R., Ingwall, J., Hale, S.L., et al. Circulation 70: 734-741, 1984.
34. Nagao, T., Matlib, M.A., Franklin, D., et al. J. Mol. Cell. Cardiol. 12: 29-43, 1980.
35. DeJong, J.W., Harmsen, E., DeTombe, P.P., Kiejzer, E. Eur. J. Pharmacol. 81: 89-96, 1982.
36. Klein, H.H., Schubothe, M., Nebendahl, K., Kreuzer, H. Basic Res. Cardiol. 74: 555-567, 1979.
37. Bourdillon, P.D., Poole-Wilson, P.A. Circ. Res. 50: 360-368, 1982.

# 17

## RECEPTORS IN THE REGULATION OF LIPOPROTEIN METABOLISM

Christopher J. Packard and James Shepherd

University Department of Pathological Biochemistry, Royal Infirmary, Glasgow G4 OSF, U.K.

Steroids play a number of important roles in human physiology. They are essential structural components of cell membranes, they act as humoral messengers, and they facilitate the digestion and absorption of dietary fat. The steroid nucleus itself comes from two sources. Approximately one half of the daily body burden of about 1.0 gm is produced endogenously while the rest is assimilated in the diet. Despite its biological indispensability, it is potentially toxic to cells if allowed to accumulate within them. Consequently, a number of mechanisms operate to regulate its intracellular concentration. This occurs at the expense of the extracellular (or plasma) pool whose mass is permitted to vary over a wide range. It is a popular misconception that the prevailing concentration of a plasma analyte is necessarily a reflection of the physiological requirement of the individual. While that may be the case for glucose or sodium, it is certainly not so for cholesterol. Animal studies have established that levels of as low as 1.0 mmol/l are adequate for the needs of the organism and many humans survive at values of 2-4 mmol/l.

In Western cultures however we have come to regard the mean population cholesterol value of about 5.5 mmol/l as "normal", even although in countries with low cholesterol levels like Japan it would be considered far from ideal. Epidemiological evidence from around the world suggests that population differences in this parameter are diet-induced. The consequence of an increased dietary saturated fat and sterol load is an expansion of the plasma cholesterol mass. Cells can sense this and reduce their sterol uptake by modulating the

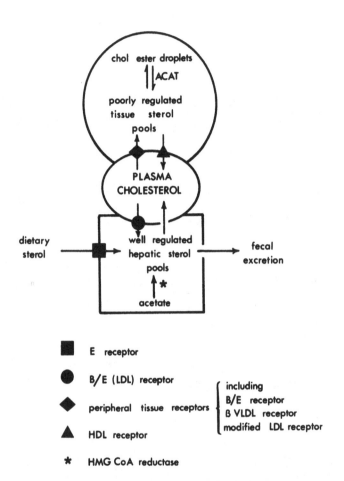

E receptor

B/E (LDL) receptor

peripheral tissue receptors { including B/E receptor B VLDL receptor modified LDL receptor

HDL receptor

* HMG CoA reductase

**FIGURE 1.** Cholesterol homeostasis in man. The liver plays a central role in corporeal cholesterol metabolism because: 1) It is the immediate destination of sterol assimilated in the diet. 2) It is responsible for the majority of endogenous sterol production. 3) It alone is capable of excreting significant amounts of the lipid. Consequently, cholesterol homeostasis within the hepatocyte is strictly regulated. Regulation of the pool occurs at the expense of the plasma compartment whose sterol level is allowed to expand under conditions of hepatic surplus. This impinges on sterol regulation at less well controlled peripheral tissue sites whose ability to exclude plasma cholesterol is limited. Excessive sterol deposition in the form of cytoplasmic cholesterol ester deposits may result in atherosclerosis. A number of cell membrane receptors have been implicated in the control of cholesterol flux between the liver and peripheral tissue pools.

activity of specific membrane proteins which serve as receptors for cholesterol-containing lipoproteins in the bloodstream. However, this process is not finely regulated in all tissues. The cells of the arterial wall, which are exposed to levels of sterol many times above that which saturates the system appear to be unable to resist influx of the sterol over the course of a lifetime. Consequently, their intracellular cholesterol pool expands and induces metabolic changes which ultimately lead to atherosclerosis. This tableau is an oversimplification of a complicated process, but does point out the pivotal role of lipoprotein receptors in regulating the balance between intracellular and extracellular sterol pools. When the process fails, disease ensues.

## CHOLESTEROL METABOLISM IN NORMAL SUBJECTS

Dietary cholesterol and triglyceride are packaged within the enterocyte to produce large triglyceride-rich chylomicron particles (for a review see Ref 1). These are hydrolysed by lipoprotein lipase in the circulation, losing in the process the bulk of their triglyceride and generating cholesterol-enriched remnants with apolipoprotein E (apo E) on their surface. This protein, the ligand for chylomicron remnant or "apo E" receptors on hepatocytes (Figure 1), triggers rapid remnant uptake by the liver, and minimises the transit time of dietary sterol through the cirulation (2). Expansion of the hepatic sterol pool leads to a number of metabolic changes. First, 3-hydroxy-3-methyl-glutaryl Coenzyme A reductase (HMG CoA reductase), the rate limiting enzyme for endogenous cholesterol production is downregulated (3). Secondly, plasma sterol assimilation via a second hepatocyte membrane receptor, the low density lipoprotein (LDL or "apo B/E") receptor, is suppressed (4). Thirdly, some of the sterol is exported into the plasma in association with very low density lipoproteins (VLDL); and finally, esterifications of a fraction of the remnant sterol results in its storage within the liver cell as relatively inert cholesteryl ester deposits. It is noteworthy that, since the liver does not possess the option of blocking remnant clearance from the plasma by downregulating chylomicron remnant uptake via the apo E receptor (5), the potentially damaging effects of these remnants on the arterial wall (see below) are obviated.

From the above description it is clear that the liver has a major influence on the level of cholesterol in the circulation. In quantitative terms, it is the most important site of lipoprotein synthesis and secretion in the post absorptive state; and in addition it harbors about 70% of LDL receptor activity in man.

The remaining LDL receptors are spread throughout the other tissues of the body some of which are also recognized to express other less well characterized lipoprotein receptor activities that may be important in modulating cholesterol balance in poorly regulated tissue pools (Fig 1), including those of the arterial wall. Their functional significance in the pathogenesis of atherosclerosis is not yet determined. Macrophages contain on their membranes a receptor (termed the beta VLDL receptor) which recognizes remnants of VLDL and chylomicron metabolism, but not LDL (6). Incubation of these cells with such remnants can induce the formation of cytoplasmic lipid droplets which may coalesce to produce a "foam" cell with the morphologic characteristics of those found in the atherosclerotic plaque. Like the apo E receptor on hepatocytes, the beta VLDL receptor of the macrophage is not downregulated in response to continuing cytoplasmic sterol accumulation. Instead, the toxic influence of this lipid is minimized by esterification, as outlined above. Unlike other cells, the macrophage is poorly endowed with LDL receptors. But, it does display high affinity for LDL whose net negative charge has been increased in a variety of ways (7). This activity also results in the generation of foam cells as the steroid pool within the macrophage expands; and it is arguable that either beta VLDL or modified LDL might be the stimulus responsible for initiating the pathogenetic process leading to atherosclerosis by permitting the accretion of cholesterol within the artery wall.

It is likely that such phenomena are continuous, even in apparently healthy arteries. Whether they result in frank pathology is probably dependent on the counterbalancing actions of mechanisms capable of re-extracting the sterol from the cells. High density lipoprotein (HDL) the smallest of the circulating lipoprotein particles, is a likely participant in this activity. Cells rich in cholesterol display HDL binding consistent with the presence of a specific receptor for the lipoprotein on their membranes (8). Such binding seems to represent a physiological process in that it fluctuates in response to changes in cellular sterol levels (8). So, the flux of cholesterol between liver, blood and peripheral tissues is governed by the integrated activities of a variety of specific protein receptors which have the potential of responding to pharmacologic agents designed to redress the imbalance in cholesterol metabolism which is thought to lead to coronary heart disease.

## INHERITED DEFECTS IN LIPOPROTEIN RECEPTOR ACTIVITY
Familial Hypercholesterolemia

The critical importance of lipoprotein receptors in human cholesterol metabolism is clearly exemplified in individuals whose inheritance of a defective gene coding for the LDL (apo B/E) receptor protein leads to atherosclerosis and premature death from vascular disease (9). The condition, familial hypercholesterolemia, is acquired by the autosomal codominant inheritance of a variety of defects within the compass of the LDL receptor gene which lead to failure of receptor-mediated catabolism of the lipoprotein. Figure 2 depicts the consequences of this defect.

Intestinal chylomicron production, intravascular lipolysis and hepatic remnant uptake are unimpaired, and so dietary sterol delivery to the liver is normal (10) - the "E" and "B/E" receptors are distinct gene products. Disruption of LDL catabolism centers largely upon the liver and results in expansion of the circulating LDL pool. This in turn redirects LDL catabolism into poorly regulated tissue pools, producing a situation in which cells like macrophages become engorged with sterol (11). Although the precise mechanism responsible for the accumulation is not known, several pathways have been proposed, including those involving the beta VLDL and modified LDL receptors described earlier. The reverse cholesterol transport system operating via the HDL receptor seems unable to compensate for this influx.

Individuals homozygous for the LDL receptor gene defect are

unable to maintain correct balance between hepatic and circulating
cholesterol compartments since, in the absence of the receptor, the
hepatocyte can neither gauge the status of the extracellular sterol
pool nor act to restore it to normal by extracting cholesterol from
the plasma and excreting it into the bile. On the other hand,

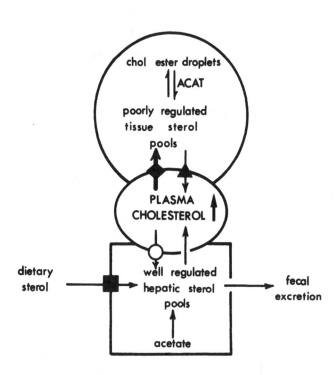

**FIGURE 2.** Cholesterol homeostasis in familial hypercholesterolemia.
Absence or deficiency of LDL (B/E) receptors on liver cell membranes
impedes the organ's ability to control the plasma cholesterol level.
The latter rises redirecting sterol into peripheral tissue pools.

heterozygous patients are able to upregulate their remaining normal
gene to advantage (12). Administration of sequestrant resins like
cholestyramine or cholestipol removes bile acids from the
enterohepatic circulation and stimulates their de novo replacement
from cholesterol. The hepatocyte responds to restore its depleted
sterol pool by:

a.  extracting LDL from the circulation

b.  increasing endogenous cholesterologenesis

So, this pharmacologic manoeuver lowers circulating LDL levels by taking advantage of the processes which maintain hepatic cholesterol homeostasis. With time, the fall in circulating LDL levels has an impact on extrahepatic tissue cholesterol pools, leading to reductions in the size of xanthomata and even to improvements in atherosclerotic arterial lesions (13). But, unfortunately, as noted above, endogenous hepatic cholesterologenesis blunts the effectiveness of treatment. However, new therapeutic agents like compactin and mevinolin, which were devised to inhibit cholesterol synthesis by inhibiting HMG CoA reductase, the rate limiting enzyme involved in the process, help counteract this escape mechanism (14).

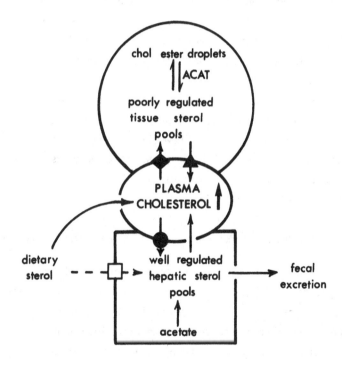

**FIGURE 3.** Cholesterol homeostasis in dysbetalipoproteinemia. This disease is characterised by defective recognition of chylomicron remnants by the apo E receptor. Dietary sterol is therefore directed into the plasma compartment and from there may be assimilated by peripheral tissues.

When administered in combination with bile acid sequestrant resins they prevent the secondary rise in cholesterol synthesis induced by the latter and produce a further increment in LDL receptor activity.

Dysbetalipoproteinemia

As indicated above, apo E on lipoprotein particles is responsible for their recognition by "E" and "B/E" receptors on cell membranes. Several common genotypic variants of this protein are found in man (15). Some compromise the ability of the protein to bind to its receptor and produce a distortion of the normal plasma lipoprotein profile. Often, this is of little consequence, but it may be brought to light by the coincident presence of a second stimulus, either genetic or environmental, which results in the appearance of frank Type III hyperlipoproteinemia. The most obvious problem in this condition is defective plasma clearance of remnants of chylomicrons and VLDL (Figure 3). In consequence, their cholesterol moiety which is normally rapidly cleared by the liver, adds to the plasma sterol pool and from there is liable to assimilation by peripheral tissue macrophages (6), producing premature severe atherosclerosis in circumstances in which circulating LDL levels are low. Obviously, nothing can be done to rectify the E protein mutation. However, it has been found that administration of estrogens (16) in these circumstances is able to reduce remnant accumulation, presumably by stimulating hepatic lipoprotein receptor activity (17).

## THERAPEUTIC MANIPULATION DESIGNED TO MODULATE OTHER LIPOPROTEIN RECEPTORS

So far we have stressed the importance of hepatic receptors in modulating plasma cholesterol pools which in turn have a secondary impact on peripheral tissue cholesterol levels. But, in theory it may be more beneficial to target therapeutic interventions against those mechanisms which govern sterol transfer between the plasma compartment and poorly regulated tissue cholesterol pools. Such agents would either limit cholesterol uptake into or promote its excretion from these pools. At the present time we do not possess compounds designed for this specific purpose, although a number of approaches are currently being made in that direction. The most promising of these involves alteration of intracellular cholesterol esterification mechanisms.

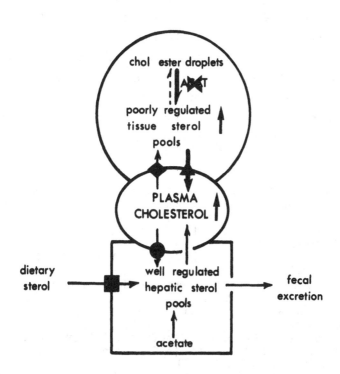

**FIGURE 4.** Acyl CoA: cholesterol acyl transferase inhibitors in the regulation of cholesterol homeostasis. It is generally accepted that peripheral tissue cholesterol accumulation predisposes to atherogenesis. Accretion of the sterol may be prevented by blocking cholesterol ester formation in peripheral tissues like the artery wall.

We have already seen that when cells accumulate sterol in excess of their requirements they can neutralise its toxic effects by esterifying it (Figure 4) via the agency of the microsomal enzyme acyl Coenzyme A: cholesterol acyltransferase (ACAT). This short term storage mechanism generates no problems in a tissue like the liver which, in times of plenty can easily excrete whatever cholesterol is surplus to requirements. However, cholesterol esterification in peripheral cells of, for example, the arterial wall has much greater potential for damage since, in this situation sterol can only be excreted in its unesterified form via the HDL reverse cholesterol transport mechanism. It follows then that agents which inhibit cholesterol esterification by blocking ACAT activity should raise free sterol levels within peripheral cells and thereby potentially improve cholesterol export by upregulating HDL receptor activity. Preliminary reports have certainly indicated that ACAT inhibition does reduce accumulation of free and esterified cholesterol in rabbit aortae (18). The clinical benefits of such interventions in man still remain to be explored.

## REFERENCES

1. Havel, R.J., Goldstein, J.L., Brown, M.S. In: Metabolic Control and Disease (Eds. P.K. Bondy and L.E. Rosenberg) W.B. Saunders, Philadelphia, p. 393-494, 1980.
2. Sherrill, B.C., Innerarity, T.L., Mahley, R.W. J. Biol. Chem. 255: 1804-1807, 1980.
3. Dietschy, J.M., Wilson, J.D. New Engl. J. Med. 282: 1128-1138; 1179-1183; 1241-1249, 1970.
4. Angelin, B., Raviola, C.A., Innerarity, T.L., Mahley, R.W. J. Clin. Invest. 71: 816-822, 1983.
5. Hui, D.Y., Innerarity, T.L., Mahley, R.W. J. Biol. Chem. 256: 5646-5655, 1981.
6. Mahley, R.W. Arch. Pathol. Lab. Med. 107: 393-399, 1983.
7. Goldstein, J.L., Ho, Y.K., Basu, S.K., Brown M.S. Proc. Natl. Acad. Sci. USA 76: 333-337, 1979.
8. Oram, J.F., Brinton, E.A., Bierman, E.L. J. Clin. Invest. 72: 1611-1621, 1983.
9. Goldstein, J.L., Brown, M.S. Ann. Rev. Biochem. 46: 897-930, 1977.
10. Goldstein, J.L., Kita, T., Brown, M.S. New Engl. J. Med. 309: 288-296, 1983.
11. Goldstein, J.L., Brown, M.S. Johns Hopkins Med. J. 143: 8-16, 1978.
12. Packard, C.J., Shepherd, J.J. Lipid Res. 23: 1081-1098, 1982.
13. Brensike, J.F., Levy, R.I., Kelsey, S.F., et al. Circulation: 69: 313-326.
14. Mabuchi, H., Sakai, T., Sakai, Y., et al. New Engl. J. Med. 308: 609-613, 1983.
15. Utermann, G., Kindermann, I., Kaffarnik, H., Steinmetz, A. Hum. Genet. 65: 232-236, 1984.
16. Kushwaha, R.S., Hazzard, W.R., Gagne, C., et al. Ann. Intern. Med. 87: 517-525, 1977.
17. Kovanen, P.T., Brown, M.S., Goldstein, J.L. Proc. Natl. Acad. Sci. USA 78: 1194-1198, 1981.
18. Bell, F.P., Schaub, R.R. Arterioscler. 6: 42-49, 1986.

# 18

## THROMBOXANE AND PROSTACYCLIN IN PLATELET/BLOOD VESSEL INTERACTION: A COMMENTARY

J. M. Ritter

Department of Clinical Pharmacology, Royal Postgraduate Medical School, Ducane Road, London W12 OHS

### INTRODUCTION

Myocardial infarction is usually caused by thrombosis in a coronary artery occurring on a ruptured atheromatous plaque, and similar pathology underlies crescendo angina and sudden ischaemic death (1). Platelets are the main cell type present in such arterial thrombi. It is also possible that platelets contribute to the development of atheroma (2,3) though this is unproven. Cyclo-oxygenase products (prostanoids) are one among several families of endogenous biologically active substances synthesised by activated platelets and damaged blood vessels which probably influence thrombosis. Whether prostanoids also influence atheroma formation is uncertain. The main cyclo-oxygenase product of platelets is the pro-aggregatory vasoconstrictor thromboxane (TX) $A_2$, while that of arteries is the anti-aggregatory vasodilator prostacyclin ($PGI_2$). Other substances produced by platelets and blood vessels which may function as mediators include platelet activating factor, nucleotides, amines and peptides. These may be at least as important as prostanoids in thrombosis. However, current interest in prostanoids is justified by clinical trials which have demonstrated that the cyclo-oxygenase inhibitor aspirin is partially effective in some vaso-occlusive disorders (4-7).

The object of this commentary is to 1) review briefly the aspects of prostanoid relevant to platelet vascular interaction; 2) consider critically the inference from clinical trials of aspirin that $TXA_2$ is important in the pathogenesis of arterial thrombosis; 3) discuss the goal of selective inhibition of cyclo-oxygenase; 4) consider the therapeutic potential of drugs acting elsewhere in the eicosanoid cascade than aspirin.

## PROSTANOID PHARMACOLOGY: PLATELETS AND BLOOD VESSELS

This subject has been comprehensively reviewed (8,9). Only the more salient points are considered here. Prostanoids are derived from essential fatty acids (see 10). These unsaturated fatty acids are present in cell membranes, esterified in the 2-position of the glycerol component of phospholipid. In Western countries the predominant fatty acid in this position is arachidonic acid, the precursor of 2-series prostanoids.

However, dietary modification can alter this situation. For instance, diets rich in oily cold-water fish are associated with increased levels of eicosapentaenoic acid, the precursor of 3-series prostanoids. In keeping with this, a metabolite of $PGI_3$ has been determined in urine of subjects eating mackeral (11) and platelets from subjects taking cod liver oil produce the weakly pro-aggregatory $TXA_3$ (12). Epidemiological data led to the hypothesis that eicosapentaenoic acid protects against thrombosis by reducing platelet aggregability (13,14). While the mechanism by which dietary eicosapentaenoic acid influences platelet function is more complex than at first thought (15,16), the possibility of favourably influencing platelet function and athero-thrombotic disease by dietary manipulation is clearly extremely attractive. Indeed, diet is one of the few interventions that could be acceptable in a general population (17).

Unsaturated fatty acid is released from membrane phospholipid by many stimuli (18,19) which include factors that may arise during the formation of an arterial thrombus such as thrombin and mechanical trauma which presumably occurs during endothelial rupture (20,21). Such stimuli activate lipases (phospholipase $A_2$, or phospholipase C and diacylglycerol lipase) which liberate free arachidonic acid. Phospholipase can be inhibited by various drugs most of which are rather non-specific (22). Phospholipase $A_2$ is also inhibited by a protein now known as lipocortin, synthesised by various cells in response to corticosteroids (see 22). Some of the profound anti-inflammatory actions of corticosteroids are probably due to this effect, which results in suppression of both cyclo-oxygenase and lipoxygenase products.    In contrast, corticosteroids do not have marked effects on haemostasis/thrombosis.  The explanation for the latter is unknown but could relate to several factors;  a) platelets are not nucleated and will therefore not themselves synthesise lipocortin in response to corticosteroids,  b) lipocortin synthesised and secreted by other cells may be rapidly diluted in circulating blood and   c) the importance of the phospholipase C pathway in platelets (23).

Prostanoids    are    synthesised    from    free    arachidonate. Cyclo-oxygenase catalyses its oxidation to $PGG_2$ and the subsequent conversion of $PGG_2$ to $PGH_2$, the common precursor of the prostanoids. Cyclo-oxygenase is inhibited by aspirin and by other non-steroidal anti-inflammatory drugs (24).  Aspirin irreversibly acetylates the enzyme (25), while drugs such as indomethacin, phenylbutazone or flurbiprofen act reversibly.  Inhibition of cyclo-oxygenase results in reduced synthesis of all prostanoids including those with opposing actions such as $PGI_2$ and $TXA_2$.  This has been referred to as the "aspirin dilemma" (26).  Strategies to achieve selectivity in the inhibition of different pools of cyclo-oxygenase in vivo are discussed below.

The fate of $PGH_2$ depends on the presence of specific synthase enzyme(s) in the cell in which is it synthesised.  Platelets contain a cytochrome P-450 enzyme thromboxane synthase which converts it to $TXA_2$ (27,28).  $TXA_2$ is formed in other organs as well as blood (e.g. lung, kidney), and by other cells as well as platelets (e.g. macrophages).

Arteries contain another cytochrome P-450 enzyme which converts $PGH_2$ to $PGI_2$ (27,29,30,31).  Vascular cells and tissues also synthesise other prostanoids as well as $PGI_2$, including $PGE_2$, $PGF_{2\alpha}$ (32,33) and even small amounts of $TXA_2$ (34), although whether this conversion occurs in vivo is still unknown.  Conversely, $PGI_2$ synthesis is not unique to vascular tissue but also occurs in pericardium, peritoneum, kidney and other structures.  $PGI_2$ escapes metabolic inactivation in the lung and it was initially thought possible that it functioned as a circulated anti-aggregatory hormone. However, the total synthetic rate of $PGI_2$ is low (35), and its concentration in blood lower than is needed to cause effects on platelets (36). It is possible to increase $PGI_2$ concentration by focal stimulation of blood vessels in vivo (37,38,39), and it is likely that it is formed and acts within the same tissue (i.e. that it is an autocoid rather than a hormone). $PGI_2$ synthase is inactivated by fatty acid peroxides (40) and it has been suggested that peroxides in atheromatous plaques inhibit $PGI_2$ synthesis in this way, contributing to the pathological process (see 41). The overall increase in $PGI_2$ synthesis reported in patients with severe atheromatous disease (42) does not preclude localized impairment of $PGI_2$ synthesis within plaques.

Imidazole inhibits thomboxane synthase (43), and more potent and specific drugs have subsequently been synthesized, including dazoxiben, dasmegrel and the Ono compounds OKY 1581 and 047. Several of these are rapidly eliminated in vivo but recently a potent thromboxane synthase inhibitor has been described which is effective for 12-24 hours in vivo in the rabbit (44). Thromboxane synthase inhibitors do not inhibit the synthesis of prostaglandins, at least at low doses, and indeed can increase $PGI_2$ synthesis by unidirectional endoperoxide diversion from platelets to endothelial cells (45,46,47). Accordingly these drugs increase excretion of the major urinary metabolite of $PGI_2$ in man (48,49).

$PGI_2$ acts on receptors that have been identified by correlation of binding characteristics with biological effects (50). The receptors activate adenylate cyclase (51,52). There is no definite evidence that $PGI_2$ receptors on different cell types (platelets, smooth muscle) differ from one another. However, no competitive antagonists of $PGI_2$ (or indeed other prostaglandins) are available, severely hindering recognition of any true differences between receptor sub-types. There are excellent competitive antagonists of $TXA_2$ (see 53) including AH 23848, BM 13177, EP 045 and SQ 29548. There are differences between the potencies of thromboxane receptor antagonists on platelets and vascular tissue, suggesting that thromboxane receptors in these tissues may differ (54,55).

## SIGNIFICANCE OF THE CLINICAL EFFECTIVENESS OF ASPIRIN

Approximately 11,000 patients with a history of myocardial infarction have been randomized in 6 published trials of aspirin. An overall analysis of outcome (a method championed by Peto of the Oxford Clinical Trials Service Unit) indicated an overwhelmingly significant improvement (22% $\pm$ 5%) in the odds of recurrence free survival in those randomized to receive aspirin (5). Smaller numbers of patients with transient ischaemic attacks have been randomized to receive aspirin but the overall results again significantly favor the drug. Two of the larger studies have been positive (3,4), although each was weakened by the use of additional drugs (sulphinpyrazone and dipyridamole respectively) which reduced the size of the aspirin only study groups. Two studies of unstable angina have shown approximately a 50% reduction of event rate in both studies (6,7). The dose of aspirin in these studies has varied from 325 mg per day to over 1 g per day without obvious differences in outcome. No studies have yet been completed using a low ("platelet selective") dose.

Aspirin prolongs bleeding time (56) and inhibits platelet aggregation induced by agonists that cause thromboxane generation (see 57 for a review). It is therefore tempting to attribute the clinical effectiveness of aspirin in preventing thrombosis to its biochemical action on cyclo-oxygenase. Such a cause-effect relationship may indeed obtain. Other explanations are however possible. Aspirin is a reactive drug and acetylates many biological macromolecules in addition to cyclo-oxygenase (58,59) and may influence the thrombotic process in ways distinct from its effect on platelets (e.g. 60). In the Canadian Co-operative Study of aspirin in patients with transient cerebral ischaemic attacks no benefit was evident in the group receiving sulphinpyrazone 200 mg 4 times daily. This dose inhibits platelet $TXA_2$ production (cf 61) although less completely than aspirin which showed significant clinical benefit in the same study (3).

The question of whether the clinical antithrombotic effect of aspirin is due to its inhibition of platelet $TXA_2$ production therefore remains open. The answer is of vital importance to antithrombotic drug development strategy. Some light will be shed on the question by studies of low dose aspirin, currently the most practicable approach to selective inhibition of platelet cyclo-oxygenase.

## SELECTIVE INHIBITION OF CYCLO-OXYGENASE

The goal of selective inhibition of cyclo-oxygenase in one cell type while sparing that in another has as its rationale the postulate that prostanoids may have deleterious effects when produced by one cell type but advantageous ones when synthesised by another. In the context of thrombosis the hypothesis might be that platelet $TXA_2$ production is harmful while the ability to synthesise vasodilator PGs in stomach, kidney and perhaps the arterial wall is beneficial. Whether this is so is unproven, but it is plausible that gastric side effects (62) and some renal side effects (63) of non-steroidal anti-inflammatory drugs would not be exhibited by cyclo-oxygenase inhibitors that spared stomach (cf BW 755C/indomethacine, 64) and kidney (cf sulindac/ibuprofen, 65) respectively. What is more controversial is whether the efficacy of aspirin could be improved by using doses that spare vascular cyclo-oxygenase (8,9,66,67,68).

Aspirin in the low dose of 0.45 mg $kg^{-1}$ $day^{-1}$ substantially inhibits platelet $TXA_2$ production (greater than 95%) without inhibiting urinary 6-oxo-$PGF_{1\alpha}$ excretion (69). Urinary 6-oxo-$PGF_{1\alpha}$ is believed to reflect renal $PGI_2$ synthesis. Whether low dose aspirin also spares vascular $PGI_2$ synthesis is less certain (70,71) especially when aspirin is given chronically (72). The argument is complicated by observations that imply that cyclo-oxygenase is synthesised more rapidly in endothelium than in deeper vascular layers (72,73). It is thus likely that in man endothelial cyclo-oxygenase is not inhibited for much of the 24 hours if it is given once daily or even more frequently (74).

The relative importance of $PGI_2$ synthesis in different vascular layers is unknown. It is probable that endothelial $PGI_2$ synthesis is important in acute thrombotic events. $PGI_2$ synthesis in the media may also be important however, perhaps by influencing the development of atheroma by effects on cholesterol metabolism (75). Further, $TXA_2$

can be synthesized in the vessel wall both by endothelium itself (34) and probably by macrophages which are an important component of atheromatous plaques ("foam cells") and which produce $TXA_2$ when stimulated (76). It is likely that a dose of aspirin that spared vascular $PGI_2$ synthesis would also spare such vascular $TXA_2$ synthesis.

Finally, it is possible that a beneficial effect of aspirin from an action on the platelet cyclo-oxygenase occurs but is a non-linear function of cyclo-oxygenase inhibition. This is rather likely to be the case because of the marked synergism between different stimuli to platelet aggregation (see 77). Furthermore, the capacity of platelets to synthesis $TXA_2$ is so much greater than the $TXA_2$ actually produced under normal or pathological conditions (78,79) even during bleeding (80). It could therefore be that while aspirin 0.45 mg $kg^{-1}$ $day^{-1}$ inhibits platelet $TXA_2$ generation by more than 95%, it still leaves enough capacity to generate $TXA_2$ that no benefit will occur in terms of inhibition of thrombosis, while the more complete inhibition caused by larger doses of aspirin (more than 100 mg/day) does have a beneficial effect.

It follows that the clinical effects of low dose aspirin cannot be predicted: it might be less effective, more effective, or equi-effective than regular dose aspirin. A comparative trial of these doses in a clinically important situation (e.g. unstable angina) will therefore be extremely interesting. Effectiveness of low dose aspirin would confirm the probable importance of platelet $TXA_2$ production in this process while greater efficacy of low dose than high dose aspirin could implicate the functional importance of $PGI_2$ or other PG synthesis. Conversely, lack of efficacy of low dose aspirin would require reappraisal of the mechanism of the anti-thrombotic effect of regular dose aspirin. The results of such a study are eagerly awaited.

## THERAPEUTIC PROSPECTS FOR OTHER DRUGS ACTING ON EICOSANOID MECHANISMS

It has been pointed out that while aspirin inhibits $TXA_2$ formation, some agonists can cause platelet aggregation by non-$TXA_2$ dependent pathways. Such stimuli include collagen, thrombin and ADP, all potentially relevant to the evolution of arterial thrombi. In contrast, $PGI_2$ inhibits aggregation irrespective of the involvement of $TXA_2$ (8,9). This makes it potentially more effective than aspirin. It might be thought that this wide spectrum anti-aggregatory action would make it dangerous. However, $PGI_2$ is relatively ineffective at inhibiting platelet adhesion as opposed to aggregation (81) and bleeding has not been a major problem in clinical practice. Indeed, $PGI_2$ has proved remarkably safe even in situations involving major surgery such as cardio-pulmonary bypass. Chemically stable analogues of $PGI_2$ (e.g. carbacyclin and iloprost) are available. However, as with $PGI_2$ itself, these analogues lack specificity for platelet as opposed to vascular smooth muscle receptors. This phenomenon renders such drugs unsuitable for long-term prophylaxis (in contrast to established short-term indications such as cardiac bypass charcoal haemoperfusion and haemodialysis).

The strategy of increasing endogenous $PGI_2$ synthesis locally at sites of vascular damage by means of a thromboxane synthase inhibitor is in theory uniquely attractive as a form of long-term treatment (cf 9). Animal data favour the notion that $PGI_2$ or thromboxane synthase inhibitors may confer greater cardiovascular protection than do cyclo-oxygenase inhibitors. Hammon and Oates (82) demonstrated that the incidence of ventricular fibrillation following circumflex coronary artery occlusion in conscious dogs was dramatically reduced by $PGI_2$ or by either of two structurally distinct thromboxane synthase inhibitors. The benefit of the synthase inhibitors was abolished by pretreatment with the cyclo-oxygenase inhibitor indomethacin. These authors drew attention to the noteworthy fact that in the AMIS trial (83) the incidence of acute myocardial infarction was reduced by aspirin, but the number of sudden deaths was greater (though not significantly greater) in the aspirin treated group. The implication is that while aspirin may have reduced the incidence of thrombosis, in fact it may have increased simultaneously the incidence of fatal arrhythmias.

Despite these and other encouraging findings on the effects of thromboxane synthase inhibitors in animal models, no clinical trials of these drugs of a size sufficient to demonstrate efficacy in thrombotic disease have been published. This situation may reflect the appreciation endoperoxide intermediates are themselves agonists at $TXA_2$ receptors (40,84). However, it is not known whether this is important in vivo. If it is so, it is probable that some strategy involving the use of drug combinations (see 85), specifically a combination of synthase inhibitor with a thromboxane receptor antagonist (86) could circumvent the problem. The existence of compounds with combined $PGI_2$ agonist/thromboxane receptor antagonist activity (87) adds an extra dimension to this possibility.

## ACKNOWLEDGEMENT

Miss Bernadette Edinborough provided expert secretarial assistance in the preparation of this manuscript.

## REFERENCES

1. Davies, M.J., Thomas, A.C. Br. Heart J. 53: 363-373, 1985.
2. Duguid, J. Path. Bact. 58: 207, 1946.
3. Ross, R. N. Engl. J. Med. 314: 488-500, 1986.
4. Canadian Co-operative Study Group. N. Engl. J. Med. 299: 53-59, 1978.
5. Editorial. Lancet i: 1172-1173, 1980.
6. Lewis, H.D., Davis, J.W., Archibald, D.G., et al. N. Engl. J. Med. 309: 396-403, 1983.
7. Cairns, J.A. N. Engl. J. Med. 313: 1369-1374, 1985.
8. Moncada, S., Vane J.R. Pharmacol. Rev. 30: 293-331, 1979.
9. Moncada, S., Vane J.R. N. Engl. J. Med. 300: 1142-1147, 1979.
10. Willis, A.L. Nutrition Rev. 39: 289-301, 1981.
11. Fischer, S., Weber, P.C. Nature 307: 165-168, 1984.
12. Fischer, S., Weber, P.C. Biochem. Biophys. Res. Commun. 116: 1091-1099, 1983.
13. Dyerberg, J., Bang, H.O., Stoffersen, E., et al. Lancet ii: 117-119, 1978.
14. Dyerberg, J., Jorgensen, K.A., Arnfred, T. Prostaglandins 22: 857-862, 1981.
15. Thorngren, M., Gustafson, A. Lancet ii: 1190-1191, 1981.
16. Thorngren, M., Shafi, S., Born, G.V.R. Br. J. Haematol. 58: 567-578, 1984.
17. Kromhout, D., Bosschieter, E.B., de Lezenne-Coulander, C. N. Engl. J. Med. 312: 1205, 1985.
18. Irvine, R.F. Biochem. J. 204: 3-16, 1982.
19. Hassid, A. Am. J. Physiol. 243: C205-C211, 1982.
20. Hong, S-C.L., Polsky-Cynkin, R., Levine, L. J. Biol. Chem. 251: 776-780, 1976.
21. Weksler, B.B., Ley, C.W., Jaffe, E.A. J. Clin. Invest. 62: 923-930, 1978.

22. Blackwell, G.J., Flower, R.J.   Br. Med. Bull.   39: 260-264, 1983.
23. Lapetina, E.G., Siess, W.  Life Sci.  33: 1011-1018, 1983.
24. Vane, J.R. Nature New. Biol.  231: 232-235, 1971.
25. Roth, G.J., Majerus, P.W.  J. Clin. Invest. 56: 624-632, 1975.
26. Marcus, A.J.  N. Engl. J. Med. 297: 1284-1285, 1977.
27. Hammarström, S., Falardeau, P.   Proc. Natl. Acad. Sci. 74: 3691-3695, 1977.
28. Ullrich, V., Graf, H., Haurand, M.  In:  Microsomes and Drug Oxidation (Eds. A.R. Boobis, J. Caldwell, F. de Mathies, and C.R. Elcombe), Taylor and Francis, London and Philadelphia, p. 95-104, 1983.
29. Bunting, S., Gryglewski, R., Moncada, S., Vane, J.R. Prostaglandins 12: 897-913.
30. Moncada, S., Gryglewski, R., Bunting, S., Vane, J.R.   Nature 263: 663-665, 1976.
31. De Witt, D.L., Day, J.S., Sonnenburg, W.K., Smith, W.L.  J. Clin. Invest. 72: 1882-1888, 1983.
32. Gerritsen, M.E., Cheli, C.D.  J. Clin. Invest.  72: 1658-1671, 1983.
33. Charo, I.F., Shak, S., Karasek, M.A., et al.  J. Clin. Invest. 74: 914-919, 1984.
34. Ingerman-Wojewsky, C., Silver, M.J., Smith, J.B., Macarak, E. J. Clin. Invest.  67: 1292-1296, 1981.
35. FitzGerald, G.A., Brash, A.R., Falardeau, P., Oates, J.A.  J. Clin. Invest. 68: 1272-1276, 1981.
36. Blair, I.A., Barrow, S.E., Waddell, K.A., et al.  Prostaglandins 23: 579-589, 1982.
37. Ritter, J.M., Barrow, S.E., Blair, I.A., Dollery, C.T.  Lancet i: 317-319, 1983.
38. Dollery, C.T., Barrow, S.E., Blair, I.A., et al.  In: Atherosclerosis: Mechanisms and Approaches to Therapy (Ed. N.E. Miller), Raven Press, New York, p. 105-123, 1982.
39. Roy, L., Knapp, H.R., Robertson, R.M., FitzGerald, G.A. Circulation 71: 434-440, 1985.
40. Salmon, J.A., Smith, D.R., Flower, R.J., et al.  Biochem. Biophys. Acta. 523: 250-262, 1978.
41. Warso, M.A., Lands, W.E.M.  Br. Med. Bull. 39: 277-280, 1983.
42. FitzGerald, G.A., Smith, B., Pedersen, A.K., Brash, A.R.  N. Engl. J. Med. 310: 1066-1068, 1984b.
43. Needleman, P., Raz, A., Ferrendelli, J.A., Minkes, M.  Proc. Nat. Acad. Sci. 74: 1716-1720, 1977.
44. Ambler, J., Butler, K.D., Ku, D.C., et al.  Br. J. Pharmac. 86: 497-504.
45. Needleman, P., Wyche, A., Raz, A.  J. Clin. Invest.  63: 345-349, 1979.
46. Schafer, A.I., Crawford, D.D., Gimbrone, M.A.  J. Clin. Invest. 73: 1105-1112, 1984.
47. Ritter, J.M.  Br. J. Pharmac. 83: 409-418, 1984.
48. FitzGerald, G.A., Brash, A.R., Oates, J.A.  J. Clin. Invest. 72: 1336-1343, 1983.
49. FitzGerald, G.A., Oates, J.A.  Clin. Pharmacol. Therap.  35: 633-640, 1984a.

50. Siegl, A., Smith, J.B., Silver, M.J., et al. J. Clin. Invest. 63: 215-220, 1979.
51. Tateson, J.E., Moncada, S., Vane, J.R. Prostaglandins 13: 389-397, 1977.
52. Gorman, R.R., Bunting, S., Miller, O.V. Prostaglandins 13: 377-388, 1977.
53. Samuelsson, B., Paoletti, R., Ramwell, P.W. (Eds.) Prostaglandin and thomboxane receptors, p. 323-358 in Advances in Prostaglandin, Thromboxane and Leukotriene Research, Vol. 11, Raven Press, New York, 1983.
54. Mais, D.E., Dunlap, C., Hamanaka, N., Halushka, P. Eur. J. Pharmacol. 111: 125-128, 1985.
55. Mais, D.E., Saussy, D.L., Chaikhouni, A., et al. J. Pharmacol. Exp. Ther. 233: 418-424, 1985.
56. Beaumont, J.L. Caen, J., Bernard, J., Sang 27: 243, 1956.
57. Weiss, H.J. Platelets. Pathophysiology and Antiplatelet Drug Therapy. Alan R. Liss, Inc., New York, 1982.
58. Hawkins, D., Pinckard, R.N., Farr, R.S. Science 160: 780-781, 1968.
59. Pinckard, R.N., Hawkins, D., Farr, R.S. Nature 219: 68-69, 1968.
60. Levin, R.I., Harpel, P.C. Weil, D., et al. J. Clin. Invest. 74: 571-580, 1984.
61. Viinikka, L., Toivanen, J., Ylikorkala, O. Br. J. Clin. Pharmac. 14: 456-458, 1982.
62. Whittle, B.J.R. In: Basic Mechanisms of Gastrointestinal Mucosal Cell Injury and Protection (Ed. J. W. Hamon), Williams and Wilkins, Baltimore, p. 197-210, 1981.
63. Clive, D.M., Stoff, J.S. N. Engl. J. Med. 310: 563-572, 1984.
64. Whittle, B.J.R. Br. J. Pharmac. 80: 545-551, 1983.
65. Ciabattoni, G., Cinotti, G.A., Pierucci, A., et al. N. Engl. J. Med. 310: 279-283, 1984.
66. Marcus, A.J. N. Engl. J. Med. 309: 1515-1517, 1983.
67. Majerus, P.W. J. Clin. Invest. 72: 1521-1525, 1983.
68. Patrono, C. N. Engl. J. Med. 310: 1326, 1984.
69. Patrignani, P., Filabozzi, P., Patrono, C. J. Clin. Invest. 69: 1366-1372, 1982.
70. Hanley, S.P., Bevan, J., Cockbill, S.R., Heptinstall, S. Lancet i: 969-973, 1981.
71. Weksler, B.B., Pett, S.B., Alonso, D., et al. N. Engl. J. Med. 308: 800-805, 1983.
72. Weksler, B.B., Tack-Goldman, K., Subramanian, V.A., Gay, W.A. Circulation 71: 332-340, 1985.
73. Frazer, C.E., Ritter, J.M. Br. J. Pharmac. in press.
74. Heavey, D.J., Barrow, S.E., Hickling, N.E., Ritter, J.M. Nature 310: 100-100, 1985.
75. Hajjar, D.P., Weksler, B.B., Falcone, D.J., et al. J. Clin. Invest. 70: 479-488, 1982.
76. MacDermot, J. Kelsey, C.R., Waddell, K.A., et al. Prostaglandins 27: 163-179, 1984.
77. Adams, G.A. In: The Platelets, Physiology and Pharmacology (Ed. G.L. Longenecker), Academic Press (London), p. 1-14, 1985.
78. Vesterqvist, O., Green, K. Prostaglandins, 27: 627-644, 1984.

79. Catella, F., Healy, D., Lawson, J.A., FitzGerald, G.A. Proc. Natl. Acad. Sci. USA 83: 5861-5865, 1986.
80. Thorngren, M., Shafi, S., Born, G.V.R. Lancet i: 1075-1078, 1983.
81. Higgs, E.A., Moncada, S., Vane, J.R. Prostaglandins 16: 17-22, 1978.
82. Hammon, J.W., Oates, J.A. Circulation 73: 224-226, 1986.
83. Aspirin Myocardial Infarction Study Research Group. J. Am. Med. Assoc. 243: 661-669, 1980.
84. Bertele, V., Cerletti, C., Schieppati, A., et al. Lancet i: 1057-1058, 1981.
85. Ritter, J.M., Dollery, C.T. Circulation 73: 240-243, 1986.
86. Gresele, P., Van Houtte, E., Arnout, J., et al. J. Thromb. Haemostas. 52: 364, 1984.
87. Armstrong, R.A., Jones, R.L., MacDermot, J., Wilson, N.H. Br. J. Pharmac. 87: 543-551, 1986.